Who Will Feed the Chickens?

Deanna Hart

National Library of Canada Cataloguing in
Publication
Hart, Deanna, 1963 –
Who Will Feed the Chickens?/ Deanna Hart
ISBN # 0-9782297-0-3

Excerpts from: *He Bear She Bear* / Stan &
Jan Berenstain, 1974; *The Unheard Cry for
Meaning* / Viktor Frankl, 1978; *Dance on
the Earth: A Memoir* / Margaret Laurence,
1989.

Cover image by Abby Selinger, copyright
2006
Typeset, printed and bound in Edmonton,
Alberta, Canada

Dhyana Body & Soul Works
12605 107 avenue
Edmonton, Alberta, Canada T5M 1Z5

for all those who are misunderstood because they suffer

for my beautiful children; Benji, Hamish and Abby

and Moscco...Sha Baby!

My Shadow

I have a little shadow that goes in and out
    with me
And what can be the use of him is more than
    I can see.
He is very, very like me from the heels up to
    the head;
And I see him jump before me, when I jump
    into my bed.

The funniest thing about him is the way he
    likes to grow -
Not at all like proper children, which is always
    very slow;
For he sometimes shoots up taller like an
    India-rubber ball,
And he sometimes gets so little that there's
    none of him at all.

He hasn't got a notion of how children ought
    to play,
And can only make a fool of me in every sort
    of way.
He stays so close beside me, he's a coward
    you can see;
I'd think shame to stick to nursie as that
    shadow sticks to me!

One morning, very early, before the sun was
    up,
I rose and found the shining dew on every
    butter-cup;
But my lazy little shadow, like an arrant
    sleepy-head,
Had stayed at home behind me and was fast
    Asleep in bed.

        -Robert Louis Stevenson

shshshshshshshshhshsh

I'm awake now. I'll do my silly arm exercises while lying here in bed. Then I'll set my feet on the floor, the rest of me still lying here, half propped up on pillows. I'll do some more exercises. Swing my arms. Press my hands together. Then ever so slowly I'll sit up, inhaling, counting to six, then exhale also to the count of six. I will stand up on another inhalation, wait till the dizziness subsides, pad into the bathroom, stick my head into the sink, turn on the taps, wash my hair, my face, twist my hair up into a towel. Look into the mirror. The spaces under my eyes will be purplish-blue, my skin pasty, but there aren't many lines even though I am now approaching forty. My body moves in slow motion. I will live to be one-hundred-twenty-six. At least. I will outlive everyone in my family, including my grandchildren. But at least they will have lived. They will have had lives to live.

I don't do this of course. I decide that it's just a waste of precious energy. It hasn't done me any good in the two years I've been practicing these wake up exercises. Instead I lie here for five more minutes, irritated that my innumerable dreams are so draining. Last night I must have begun to feel nauseated in my sleep again and it was incorporated into my dream. People were vomiting everywhere and I kept pouring bottles of Gravol tablets into my mouth but couldn't swallow. By the time I shook myself awake it was too late. But I managed to drift off again sometime before my alarm woke me once more. Now my stomach feels numb, which is good. Numb is good.

1

I drag myself from my bed, throw my bathrobe over my shoulders, stumble into the bathroom, pour bath water as hot as I can stand it, plunk myself into the tub to ease out some of the painful stiffness. I swear, some days, that rigor mortis is setting in a little prematurely. I wash my hair, pull the plug, pat myself dry, twist my hair into a towel around my head. I don't bother looking into the mirror. I know what's there. And what isn't.

I flip the kitchen light on, rinse a pot and pour in some tap water and salt, turn a burner on to maximum. No lunches made last night, I see. I must have forgotten again. And heaven forbid that the kids should actually do anything of their own accord, at least not without being told a dozen times. So I defrost a couple slices of bologna, smear mustard and mayonnaise onto four slices of bread, slap on the half-cooked bologna, some lettuce, slice them into two, wrap in plastic, stumble to the stove, pour rolled oats into the boiling water, turn down the burner. It boils over anyway.

Then I wake up the kids. They growl at me, pull the covers up over their heads, tell me to go away and turn off the light.

I can't, I say. *It's not my fault you have to get up in the morning and go to school. It's only my fault you were born and it's too late to have an abortion.* But they are never amused at six-forty-five a.m.

Somehow the porridge gets eaten, the lunches get packed, mismatched socks get put on, coats get found, notes get signed, money gets handed out to avoid an argument, the door gets slammed, homework gets left behind, but at least they're gone and I topple back into bed.

I read for a bit until the words mutate into black bugs crawling over the pages. Drowsiness overcomes me like a sheet of lead. I will pull my pillows down, wrap myself in the blankets. I will close my eyes and watch the insides of my eyelids until the tunnels appear and then I will float into the tunnels. My body will begin descending, sinking, and then will plummet sharply till I hit bottom. The bottom is a wonderful

2

place to be, confusing sometimes, but now that I have begun to understand and master these episodes, I can usually control where I go, how it feels and when I wake. These are my only moments of reprieve.

But I don't have time to consider what will happen this time. Instead, I find I am beginning to arouse, ascending from sleep, up from the bottom, back into my body, into full awareness. I don't want to move. Complete relaxation has stilled every cell and I glance groggily at the clock. It has only been fifteen minutes, maybe less. As I lie here tangled in my blankets, my mind replays the last vivid fifteen minutes, though it seemed like hours, days even.

First I watched my eyelids, perhaps only for a few seconds this time. Thoughts meandered through my mind but I swept them away, like dust. Poof. Within only a few minutes, I felt the thud of my consciousness hit bottom and knew I was asleep. I opened my eyes, as I usually do, and watched the rest of my body lying there, so still you'd think it was dead. My conscious mind was detached from my limbs and trunk and the sensation of nothingness was ethereal compared to the ache and intense drowsiness only moments before. I tried to remain in this state, but my auditory senses were playing tricks on me again. This time I heard the cats, not meowing, not purring, but screeching right inside my ears. I tried to lift my arms to calm them, tried to speak to them, but my body was paralyzed. I couldn't move, no matter how hard I willed myself to move, turn over, wake from the hallucination. Then I remembered I was only asleep. The cats were outside. I had closed the door. I was asleep. There were no cats. No screeching. Nobody but me and my breath.

Then there were the tunnels again, twisting, spinning, like the tunnels you read about in near-death experiences, and I was cruising down the center of a spiral at the speed of light, maybe faster. The sensation was hypnotizing. I tried to propel myself to the end this time, but suddenly there was my daughter, at the door, asking for some ice cream, and the television was on, blaring the Flinstones' theme song. But so loudly. I was annoyed that they wouldn't turn it down, knowing their mother was sleeping. So I sat up to squawk at her. But my eyes opened again, and there was no little girl standing in the doorway, and I had not sat up. The music must have been an hallucination too. It always is.

That's what I told myself as my mind focused again on the motionlessness of my body under the blankets. The utter and complete relaxation. Every muscle, every pore, every hair absolutely still. I wanted to stay there. This is my secret nirvana.

But here I am again, thinking it through. Contemplating. Wondering. Feeling alone because no one else I know experiences these things.

You should be assessed for narcolepsy is what some doctors have suggested. But what would be the point in knowing for sure I have narcolepsy? The treatment is an indefinite course of amphetamines, which my stomach and nervous system would not appreciate.

I used to cry, before I learned to accept and understand these hypnotic sleeps. My precarious emotions would escalate, then topple over each other landing in a muddled heap. The individuation of mind and body would create a heightened mental and emotional awareness and leave me detached from my own body. I would feel frightened. Powerless. Calm. Bewildered. Crazy. And alone. In the summers I would go down to the dock, toss a handful of pellets to the fish. I would talk to them. In the winter I would pull on my snow suit and boots, wrap my head like a mummy in scarves, and walk until the heaviness returned, then stumble home, every bone aching, every muscle exhausted, every vein weary with defeat.

Now I just smile to myself. There is no one around to smile at. Sometimes I smile in the mirror, my fingers tracing where the lines should be around my eyes and mouth. I look twenty-three years old, not thirty-five. It's deceptive - the way I look. People look at me and sneer,

But you look so healthy, is what they say to me. To each other they whisper, *she's just making it up. There's nothing*

wrong with her. She just wants attention, and by golly, we're not giving it to her. She's crazy. Loonier than a cuckoo.

Sometimes, like today, I roll over and go back to sleep. A dreamless, uneventful sleep this time. Another hour rolls by. When I wake, there is no pain. I feel groggy, but peaceful, okay. It is only ten o'clock. If I hurry I can get dinner into the slow cooker and some laundry done before the crash. If I'm careful not to eat I might be able to get through the morning and part of the afternoon. But it takes such discipline to stay away from the fridge. I get so hungry that I become frantic, shaky.

Hypoglycemia, some doctors say. *Eat frequent small meals. Avoid the low sugar levels. Trust me, you'll feel better.* But labels don't make any difference. Eating makes me lethargic, bloated and sore all over. So I would rather be frantic and shaky than in pain.

But first I roll out my yoga mat, stretch out the stiffness again. I would like to study yoga. Not just the postures. I'd like to study the science of yoga. Mind over matter. With proper breathing, I've read, one can control all of one's physical matter. One can achieve ultimate bliss. No pain. No fatigue. Nothing but pure bliss. One day I will be well enough to travel to India, study with a master. I will learn to concentrate, meditate. I will learn to control bodily sensations, functions. I will be without pain because I will have learned to think the pain away. I will have worked my inner organs into submission. My body will work for me, with me, not against me.

I have an overabundance of time because of this condition. And so I read a whole lot. My concentration is poor. Brain fog heavy. Nevertheless, I do manage to ingest copious amounts of book knowledge while ordinary people have to work for a living. I am partial to Canadian writers of course. I have read everything Margaret Laurence ever wrote at least three times over. Her women are genuine, down to earth and full of marvelous cynicism. Margaret Atwood's women are insolent egomaniacs and I adore them all. I am

5

currently reading a new Canadian author, Gail Anderson Dargatz. Her photograph is on the back inside cover. I see that she was born in 1963, the same year my mother gave birth to me. Her brief biography tells me she has a life. I wonder what that would be like. To have a life.

I also read American novelists. Hemingway and Fitzgerald I don't particularly care for, but Kurt Vonnegut Jr.'s schizophrenic reasoning appeals to my sense of deranged idealism. Most of all I like his hairdo.

I read other books too. Religious books of all kinds. Hindu scriptures; Buddhist; the Tao Te Ching; the Bible of course; philosophers galore, though sometimes I think philosophy too personal, almost like watching someone bathe; psychology textbooks; cookbooks about cheese-making, gourmet meal planning, etc; books on frogs, flowers, boreal forests, and whatnot.

I don't talk much. Not out loud. There doesn't seem to be enough air in me. But it's just as well because nobody really wants to talk to me anymore. Most of the people I know, including some family members who I won't name, have decided I'm too stuck up for words, or that I'm some kind of *voodoo zombie, mostly gone. She's not quite all there,* I've heard said. Or, *is she okay in the head? I wonder why her husband stays with her. Those poor children,* and so on.

It's alright though. Other than gossip, I've realized that most of these people out here in the country only want to talk about Pic seed and John Deere tractors. And each other. Lots of them talk about money, a subject that does not interest me at all.

The Bible tells me that if one can curb his tongue, then the whole body is under control and he is a fully developed character, perfect, and able to control his entire nature.

I can do a headstand now. It's a new posture I've been working on. I still have to use the wall for support and sometimes my head threatens to explode. But if conditions are right, it seems to stabilize my blood pressure and I will feel refreshed, clearer, and breathing seems easier, fuller, more complete. I've all but given up recording my daily blood pressure as my doctor wishes me to do. It never changes much, ranges between about 70/45 all the way up to 95/60. Some doctors have told me it's *a blessing in disguise. Low blood pressure is associated with longevity, very slim risk of developing heart disease or stroke.* They think they are presenting me with a pleasing prognosis, as though longevity is an elusive state to be desired, worshipped almost, and I should be thrilled. Medical nirvana maybe. Personally, I think thirty-five years are plenty.

There. A complete cycle of sun salutations and I'm not shaking. In fact, one could say I almost feel good. What does it really mean to feel good? I doubt that I have a decent sense of objectivity in this regard. I'm standing. My stomach only hurts a little. My fingers and feet are freezing, but they are only small appendages. No vital organs are contained in them. My heart is thrumping in its peculiar, irregular way, which makes me feel lightheaded, but the world is not turning black and my eyesight is nearly perfect.

I would love a cup of Red Rose tea right now. With a swirl of milk and a teaspoon of sugar, steaming hot, bordering on burning my tongue, rolling down my throat. I would cradle the cup with both hands, fingers interlocked, feeling the heat steep right through my frigid fingers. But eventually it would hit my stomach, which would revolt upon contact.

So I sweep the tea thought from my mental theatre and replace it with a piece of dry toast which still looks rather delectable as long as I don't get carried away and have two pieces which I sometimes, regretfully, do. Or spread margarine on it as I have also done and regretted. This is alright with me too, for I have read in some of my philosophy books that attachment to worldly or sensual pleasures only leads one further away from achieving true Nirvana. I have also read that in a person's final cycle of Samsara, he or she will begin to live the life of a recluse, without attachments or desire to lead him or her astray. (All the books say *him,* I have added the *her.*

I'm certain that the author didn't intend any gender discrimination as most of these writings were set down in earlier centuries and gender pronoun usage had not yet become politically censored).

I do try to keep up some sort of social life, though it is more for my husband's and children's sake. I have become more of an observer than participant. Three or four times a year the community throws together a dinner and dance and tacks on a title like, *Fall Wild Game Supper*, or *News Year's Eve Dance*, or *An Evening of Cowboy Poetry*. No one can appreciate the preparation it takes for me to attend one of these functions. A few days beforehand I will start taking sleeping medication in the afternoon and at night, sort of like a camel stocking up on water. I will fast on the day of the feast and stay in bed all day except for a couple of hot baths and a few yoga stretches. I must dress warmly because most of these people are smokers and all of the doors remain open in spite of -20C temperatures.

Last November I contributed a pot of trout chowder to the wild game supper. I'm sure that if anyone had known who made it, they wouldn't have touched it. But my beautiful pot of chowder sat steaming on the long central table anonymously and was devoured before half the party had eaten their way through the line.

I can sit well enough as long as there is something to support my elbows. I can even dance. Clear the dance floor for me during the polka! As long as I'm moving I'm okay. But standing in line is another thing altogether. I asked my doctor why such a simple non-activity would cause such horrendous physical distress.

When you're moving around, she says, *the blood is circulating. When you're just standing still, the blood pools in your legs, oxygen is not getting to your brain, your blood pressure drops and you faint. Know your limits and don't overextend them. Always carry a camping stool with you. Sit down.*

I don't, of course. Their loose tongues wag quite enough

around here. I try to be inconspicuous but am almost never successful at this.

These events are like carnivals to me. Better than Halloween. Costumes more vivid, colorful, amazing. You'll never see so many racy western shirts, gaudy belt buckles and star-spangled wallets as you'd see at the community hall on a dance night. Some of the men even wash their hair, or at least comb it. I don't usually recognize them without their farmer caps on, so it's like seeing a brand new bunch of people. The women bustle about in the kitchen, their thighs swishing together in tight jeans, heels clacking against the cold linoleum floor. The men buy drinks for one another and guffaw a whole lot, running their fingers through their sparse hair.

The fusion of voices, smoke and halitosis is almost fatal and I find myself wandering around outside every half-hour or so. I don't speak with anyone. My voice is not strong enough to carry through smog and noise, viscous as castor oil. This is all right with me though because I am rarely spoken to. I prefer to listen, catch up on all the local gossip. When my husband is with me, everyone at the table chatters and guffaws. When he goes for another drink or a bathroom break, there is a conspicuous deadlock at our table until his return.

I only wanted to stand in line like everyone else, fill my plate with a baked potato and sour cream, maybe some salad with no dressing, a bun without butter. My mouth had been watering all day, preparing for that moment, the moment which I would savor slowly, purposefully chewing each mouthful of food that I hadn't had to cook, swallowing with the slow anticipatory deliberation of one approaching ecstasy.

My husband was behind the bar, serving drinks. My kids were being pests somewhere. And there I was, standing in line, holding my plate and my plastic fork and knife, waiting. Waiting. Standing. And then my knees began to wobble. I felt that irregular rhythm of my heart, pounding, crashing against my chest, in my throat, squeezing my brain, emptying it of oxygen. I tried to suck a deep breath in like I usually do when this happens, counting to six. But by count three, I noticed that the nice lady behind me, bless her, had courteously moved aside so that nothing would impede my speedy gravitation to the floor.

That's all I remember until I looked up into my husband's mutating face and he had his big burly hands against my cheeks saying that I felt cold and clammy. I waited until his face stopped appearing and dissolving, and began to solidify, then I said, *that's because you've laid me in the snow again.* And he laughed at me, picked me up till my feet were dangling off the ground and squeezed me so tight I almost fainted again.

Are you okay now? Do you want me to take you home?

Of course not. Put me down.

Aren't you wearing your heart monitor? Why aren't you wearing it? You could've sat down in time. I should've been with you. Do you want me to come sit with you?

No, Silly. Go away. I'm fine. I'm hungry.

And so he butted in line, returned with my potato and salad and bun and some goopy saskatoon-berry stuff, kissed me, and strutted back to the bar and I savored the food that I had waited for all day. It didn't matter much to me that one of my relatives, whose name I won't mention, was across the hall whispering into the ears of another gawk-eyed listener. My son brought his plate, heaped with steaming elk sausage, venison chili, bear stew, ostrich patties, and marshmallow salad, and sat down next to me.

Are you okay, Mom? You should be the stunt-Mom of the year. Super Dave Mom.

I remember the first time. The warm, humid, early spring scent still clings to my memory like the dew of that morning. If you could take the air and wring it out, there would have been a heavy downpour that day. But the moisture was unconsolidated, everywhere; on the ground, resting heavily on the purple crocuses which were sprinkled sparsely over the prairies, valiantly peeking through the few remaining crusts of snow; pussy willows shimmering like drops of silver; barren limbs of poplars and alders, dark and weighted with moisture; the mossy shingles of our aging farmhouse roof beginning to separate and lift. Gray clouds hung over the earth, shielding it from the sun, allowing the earth a long replenishing drink after the winter's deep slumber.

It was a beautiful grayness. Beautifully haunting. I felt disconcerted like something inside me was becoming disconnected from itself. At any moment I could become unstuck and go floating off into space without even the assurance of an orbit to follow. There was only one of me. Only one. I remember thinking too, that there was only one of God. And only one devil. Just the three of us. The rest of humanity got lumped into a collective heap of unimportance.

I had not slept well the last couple of nights. I had lain awake, listening to the eerie cry of coyotes in some distant coulee, my father's habitual snoring seeping up through the heat ducts, a few scattered drops of rain pattering against the roof. Comforting nighttime sounds. By early morning I would doze off only to be awakened by my mother banging pots and pans together down in the kitchen.

That morning she came into my room, flicked on my bedside lamp as she usually did, and began to caress my forehead, gently stroking my damp hair away from my face. But I couldn't open my eyes. I seemed to be shrouded in a vague, shadowy fog. My limbs felt heavy, my bones beginning to petrify.

You feel a little warm, Honey, she whispered touching the back of my neck. *Aren't you feeling well today?*

Sleepy, is all I could murmur.

She placed both hands on my cheeks, then on my forehead. *Is your throat sore?* Tender concern in her voice.

A little.

Maybe you should stay home for a day, stay in bed. Do you want to stay home?

I shook my head side to side on the pillow. *No.*

Well come on down then and I'll fix you some hot tea for

your throat. Dress warm, it's a little drizzly today. I won't have you catching a chill.

She patted my shoulder, brought my bathrobe and slippers and padded back down the stairs. Even back then I wasn't comfortable with an excess amount of attention. I preferred to blend in, a conscious effort on my part. I loved my mother's gentle-hearted caresses and tender words, but I did not want to be fawned over or noticed in any distinct way. And so I dressed, sipped her tea, declined breakfast, tucked my thermos of soup under my arm and plodded on down the driveway to wait for the school bus.

My insides felt queasy, all tangled and pulled up into knots. My throat was swollen, sinuses congested, but not bad enough to warrant a day in bed. I rarely missed school. If I was ill, I was ill only on weekends and always recuperated in time for my mother's scrumptious Sunday pot roast. I do not believe that I was ever spoiled despite being an only child. Both my parents were gentle and compassionate, though my mother was more outspoken than my loveably reserved, father. There was no reason in the world why I should have felt the neglect, the insecurity and anxiety I was feeling that dismal gray morning. I tried humming it away, inventing tunes of my own, stories to go with the tunes, but soon fell silent.

School that morning was uneventful. Our sixth-grade teacher had a voice that sounded like sandpaper felt against your skin. He was frightening to look at too; sunken cheeks, dark wiry mustache half-concealing thin, waxy lips; beady, depthless eyes; and that cologne-coated musty odor that seeped from his skin. I did my work studiously and quietly, not to avoid personal confrontation with him, but to avert the smell and grating voice. Perhaps I was overly sensitive even then.

At lunchtime the country students filed into the assembly room where we would open our lunch boxes after prayer, eat, giggle, kick each other, poke fun at the stinky kid, and fantasize about the dreamboat drama teacher. But that particular day I only wanted to be alone. I didn't want anyone pestering me with irrelevant questions.

Why aren't you eating your lunch? Do you want some of my peanut butter sandwich? Isn't he cute? I didn't feel ill exactly, just not quite well, and it was nobody's business.

Some of the other girls had already started their cycles. They said sometimes, that they didn't feel well. Sometimes it hurt. *I got cramps today,* one of the girls would groan emphatically in the gym change room, clutching her lower abdomen, doubling over, and all of the other girls would groan too and pat her on the shoulders, exchange sympathetic looks, and argue over who would carry her gym bag, and one would even offer to keep an eye on the back of her dress. Having one's period, it appeared, subjected one to excess attention, poking and prodding, responding to embarrassing questions and allowing oneself to be on a kind of ceremonious display. Therefore, I was dreading the inevitable and it had crossed my mind that, perhaps, this ill feeling of late was an indication that my girlhood was coming to an end. If so, I would have to devise a plan of guarding secrecy for as long as possible.

My hands were beginning to tingle, then my legs. A strange, dizzying whirring sound was coming from the inside of my ears, inside my head. I had to get out of there in a hurry but it was only twelve-twenty. Lunchroom teacher didn't dismiss us until twelve-thirty. I replaced the lid of my thermos, soup untouched. I could ask to be excused to go to the bathroom but I had never made such a request in all my years at school. It was nobody's business if I had to go to the bathroom, and I would hold it, even if it meant a bursting bladder, until recess. I should have accepted my mother's offer to stay home. What if something red appeared on the back of my dress and everybody saw it? Or worse, what if I threw up? I couldn't wait. I would raise my hand, just like anybody else would have and ask to go to the bathroom. Just this once. But where had my hands gone? Those two listless appendages were hanging, almost numb, at my side. Where was my side? Where were my feet so that I might just get up and run out without asking permission? All at once my left arm thrust itself out before me to keep the floor from rising up and

13

smacking me in the face.

Next thing I knew, my mother was leaning over me with a paper bag of jelly donuts under her arm, stroking my hair and chanting my name. It appeared that I was lying on a cot in the school infirmary, amidst the pungent odor of Pine Sol and rubbing alcohol. The lunchroom teacher was also hovering over me, explaining to my mother what must have happened. He sounded apologetic, alarmed.

She just fell out of her chair. I heard a thump, looked up, and there she was, sprawled out on the floor. She never said anything at all. I think she might have hit her head, there's a lump there on the side of her forehead, see.

My mother swept my bangs back, felt the contours of my forehead with her cool fingertips. *Honey? Are you all right? You fainted.* The first sensation that swept through my thought files was relief. Relief that my mother had come and could whisk me away from this sick-smelling place, away from the curious stares of my classmates, which precipitated the second sensation - humiliation. Floods of humiliation, more overpowering than the feelings of fright and anxiety that had been hanging over me the last few days. I could never go back to class now. They would all be hovering about, touching me, asking me how I felt, what was wrong, did I feel better, did I have to go to the hospital, would it happen again, and so on.

I suppose then, that my eyes began to get watery, my nose red and runny, for my mother, whose remedy for every ailment was food, held out the bag of jelly donuts.

Here, I brought donuts - raspberry, lemon, blueberry, and I think a chocolate glaze too. You didn't eat much today. It's no wonder. And then turning to the teacher, she continued, *it's no wonder she fainted. This girl has been eating like a bird lately. Not a single bite for breakfast, and not much for supper last night either, if anything at all. It's no wonder.*

Let's get you home and feed you, she said to me, offering her hand to help me up.

I was still shaking, more from embarrassment than lightheadedness, so I accepted her gesture. The teacher stepped aside, my mother's arm around my shoulder, me clutching the bag of donuts. We collected my jacket and boots from the hallway and boot room, then my mother guided me gently into the front seat of our eggshell Plymouth station wagon.

You wait right here, Honey. I'm just going to have a word with your teacher. I'll be right back. Why don't you nibble on a donut? You'll be better in no time.

I knew what she'd say. She'd tell him I would be away for a few days, maybe a week, until I was fattened up and rosy again. She'd ask for some homework. She'd probably tell him to lighten up on the students, not push them so hard. She would probably mention that I had never had the measles or mumps, but that she thought I'd had chicken pox as a baby, and that I was hardly ever ill and did not like to miss school and deserved a few days of rest. She wouldn't say all these things quietly in the privacy of a hallway corner. No, she would waltz right into the classroom, announcing her presence with the clip-clop of her heels and the polished stride of a model. She would look him straight in those beady eyes and speak to him with the grace of a queen and the authority of a military general. The other children would become hushed, stricken with awe and envy. When I did return to school I would have to endure unbreathable attention for this. But never mind all that, a taste of lemon jelly donut was beginning to stir, then calm, those rumblings in my stomach and I began to feel steady again, safe, less evasive, solid.

The door opened and my mother appeared laden with textbooks, notebooks and pencil crayons, which she set into a semi-ordered heap between us.

Feeling better now? I just figured you'd need a few days work sent home. I told him I wasn't going to send you to school until we fattened you up and put some color back into those cheeks. You've never really been sick a day in your life, except for the chicken pox when you were a baby and that only lasted a couple of days, if that. Never had mumps or measles or anything I told him. A couple days off school won't hurt.

Do you some good.   I think he works those kids too hard sometimes, don't you?   I told him so too, right in front of everybody.

That was the first time.

Shshshshshshshshshshsh

(I married an angel. I didn't know it at the time, but I know it now. I'm thinking this in parentheses, in whispers, because I am afraid that if God knows I know, He'll take my angel away from me. I would never voice this to anyone. Not anyone, not even God. Especially God. There is something very ethereal, fearfully sacred, about being married to an angel of course. One always has to take utmost care in treating one's angel with impeccable respect and consideration. Once, I thought my guardian angel had moved on until I realized that my own spouse had become my angel, or my angel had become my spouse.

He even has an angel's name. He looks something like Michelangelo's David, only a little taller, shoulders a little broader. Just to throw me off a little, he was endowed with a few human qualities, like amnesia. My beloved gets amnesia daily. But he only forgets the things that don't need to be remembered. I suppose it is like that in heaven, where he is from. I take that back, about amnesia being a human quality. Humans forget the good things and remember the bad. My angel doesn't seem to know that evil exists in this world. To him all things are good.

The other human quality is that he is a diabetic. Every day I watch him pierce his body with those needles, three a day, in his thigh, in the micro-inch of fat on his belly or his butt. Without those needles he would not be here. Without him, where would I be? The needles make him human. The

17

needles make him understand me).

God must accept me. He has to. The Bible says that I am sanctified by my believing husband. I don't know that I am exactly unbelieving. I believe in a lot of things. I believe that we are real. We are not just illusions living on an illusive time line. But I also believe in illusions. I believe we all need our illusions to cope with all of our various perceptions of reality. I believe in treating all of God's creatures with dignity and respect, although a great many of God's creatures don't seem to share that belief. I believe in gardens even though I can't seem to grow one. I believe that puppies are the antidotes to just about all of our physical and mental infirmities, in much the same way that my mother believed in the healing power of food, especially jelly donuts. I believe in the universal law of gravity and Kepler's three laws of planetary motion even though I am not a mathematician, although I am a pseudo-scientist of sorts. Science is the most beautifully written poetry as far as I'm concerned. I do prefer evidence, though there usually isn't any for the things that I would like to believe.

Like this:

I also believe that I am well. Somewhere inside, inside this boundless inner-space in which my Self is contained, I know that I am well. Somehow I have let my body take control of my mind. But I do have the knowledge, the capacity, and the power to reverse that control. We all do. But where is it? How?

I also believe in suicide, though the very word connotes sadness, unnecessary tragedy. It shouldn't. If an individual has become so despondent with living that the only relief seems to be in non-living, then for Pete-on-a-pogo-stick's sake, why not? One of the most absurd human indecencies I have ever witnessed was a ninety-eight-year old man being forced to swallow antidepressants because he'd had enough living.

I have to stop and think about this for a moment. You are ninety-eight years old. You have lived your life. You have worked, raised a family, seen the technological world transform from authentic horsepower to machine power. You have been through two wars, at least. You have watched both your parents die, your brothers and sisters also, one at a time, probably even one or two of your children, maybe even a grandchild or great-grandchild. You are the only one left. You alone remain to count out your days in a foul-smelling nursing home where you are paraded around in diapers, wheelchairs and walkers; forced to endure polkas and waltzes and accordions and well-meaning reverends who come in once a month to spread one last word to the sick and dying; one by one your old chums are carted off to the hospital and they don't return, their names quietly erased from the placemats on the dining room tables; if you are agile enough, you play shuffle board, if not, you watch censored movies; you are spoon-fed and sometimes you have accidents in your pants and stink up the whole ward; what you remember of your life is spoken of in past tense, although there is rarely occasion to speak of it, and what remains now is a daily dose of vivid mortifications.

When the mind has had enough living for one lifetime, the body will quickly follow. This is the natural course of a life span. To tinker with nature is an open invitation for misery. Let them go and let them go peaceably and respectably is what I say.

There are other, justifiable, reasons to end one's own life. Other than old age I mean. For instance, I hold utmost admiration and respect for Margaret Laurence, who rationally and methodically plotted out her final days and hours. When it became apparent that she might outlive her charted course due to breakthroughs in modern medicine, and in those extra days or months, would be incapacitated to the point where total palliative care would be the only viable way through, she decided to unburden her family by taking matters into her own hands. She recorded the minutes leading up to the event with thoughtful precision. She was smart. She did not want anyone to have to deal with the mess of a failure so she swallowed anti-emetics before the deadly ingestion.

I love Margaret Laurence. *Peggy*, is how I think of her. I converse with her sometimes. *Peggy and I. Me and Peggy.*

Her grandfather called her Peggy also.

Peggy writes in her memoir, *real people are more important than writing; life is always more important than art.* I ask her about this statement sometimes.

Whatever can you mean by that, Peggy?

And she answers me,

Real people are the stuff of writing. There would be no story without the re-creation of real people into fictional form. You observe, you listen, you feel. Real people make you You. Fictional people make you somebody else. Art is the representation of yourself and your perception of your world. It is merely form, and only two-dimensional. People are multi-dimensional, and not limited to form.

But why do we persist in re-creating ourselves? Why do we want distortions of what we perceive as reality?

Because, she answers with amused patience, *perceptions of reality are also multi-dimensional and as diverse and varied as snowflakes. Art draws forth those vast and infinite perceptions.*

I'm not so sure. Maybe I read too much. Maybe I drool over photographs of Good Housekeeping casseroles more than I should. I get confused, think I am part of the picture, or the story. It's hard to distinguish, sometimes, the art, the fictional, the unreal, from what's real. I don't particularly like real people. I like made-up people much better. The people I create are much nicer to me. They don't scoff or whisper rude things when they think I can't hear because sometimes I am invisible. My people are kind. They don't ostracize me for my weaknesses. They understand. They even offer support and comfort. They don't make me want to disappear. I prefer to live in my paintings, my pictures on the wall and in magazines, and in the words of my books.

Peggy is beautiful. She resembles Toad in Wind in the Willows. But that is only my perception. Perhaps she really looks like Mole, or Ratty. Who is to say?

Peggy also describes her inner battle over her work - her writing - and her marriage. Ultimately her writing took front seat. When my children were young I used to read a book to them, entitled, "He Bear She Bear". Mother and Father bear are instructing their bear children on the near-infinite career possibilities awaiting them as big bears. It is as simple as a choice. The indoctrination goes like this:

> *We could fix a clock*
> *paint a door*
> *build a house*
> *have a store*
> *drive a truck*
> *drive a train*
> *bulldoze roads*
> *drive a train.*
> *We do all these things, you see*
> *whether we are he or she...*
>
> *You could be a doctor*
> *make folks well*
> *teach kids how*
> *to add and spell*
> *knit a sock*
> *sew a dress*
> *paint a picture*
> *what a mess!*
>
> *You could lead a band*
> *sing a song*
> *play a tuba*
> *beat a gong*
> *play a banjo*
> *plink-a-plink.*
> *You could even play*
> *on a kitchen sink...*
> *I may build bridges*

I may climb poles
I may race cars
I may dig holes
I could be a magician
I could go on TV
I could study the fish
who live in the sea.
I'll be a cowboy
I'll go to the moon
I'll feed a whale
I'll train a baboon
We'll fly a giant jumbo jet
We'll build the tallest building yet
We will jump on a trampoline
We'll tame twelve tigers
and twenty-six fleas
We'll do a dance on a flying trapeze
We'll jump and dig
and build and fly
There's NOTHING that we cannot try!

Why are we not taught the impossibilities? So many things I wanted to do and be. When I was young I thought I wanted to be a school teacher; then an artist; then a nurse in a third world country where I would tend to my patients with tireless devotion; then a professional gardener with acres and acres of lush berries and warm, steamy greenhouses; then a flight attendant who traveled the world; then a beekeeper so that I could wear a white suit and netted helmet and play with bees that flow through your fingers like the honey the produce; then a marine biologist on an offshore laboratory. When I was older, in high school, I thought about being a chemist, mad with ideas, discoveries; a clinical psychologist who made people well by listening to them; then a truck driver chaining up my tires for a descent down snowy passes; then a forester; then a potter; a fashion designer; or maybe a social worker; an auto mechanic and so on.

> *So many things to do and be*
> *whether we are he or she.*

Instead, these things turned out to be a list of impossibilities, the things I could not do or be.

So you see, Peggy, for some of us, the unreal is much more pleasant, more viable, more real.

This is one of the things in which I believe the most. Delusions.

My husband tells me that I am good. *Good,* he says, like good is something esteemed, a virtue that eradicates all other flaws. If you are good, it is all right to be ugly, for instance. Or, if you are good, you can be stupid and nobody will take notice. You could be a lousy cook or have no musical ability whatsoever or forget to shut off the water valve while watering the horses so that the well runs dry and you will be forgiven because, after-all, you are *good.* Or you could be weak and sickly so that most days all you can do is drag yourself from the bedroom to the bathroom to the kitchen and then back to the bedroom; your children must sneak around the house so they don't disturb you and they can never have friends in; their teachers think you are an alcoholic or have some sort of mental illness because you often forget to sign their notes and you rarely answer the phone and when you do, your voice crackles so that you sound like you have a hangover or you've been sleeping for one hundred years; your husband entertains his few guests outside or on the verandah so they don't intrude, but guests are a rare occasion because they've all heard about you, the eccentric wife, and your bizarre behaviors, thanks to a particular relation who isn't really worth mentioning; sometimes dinners aren't on time; all the windows are covered in fly specks, fingerprints and paw-marks galore; cobwebs are strung from the fan to the ceiling; gobs of dust and lint fill every corner. See, all these shortcomings are magically blotted out if you are *Good.*

Good is merely the other side of Bad. We recognize Good only in its relation to Bad. The human condition must be in a constant state of conflict over which side of the stick is up and which is down.

Wilma was Good. I loved Wilma. I love her still though I don't know where she is. I heard that she went back to Pennsylvania where she is working as a nurse. This would seem sensible, as Wilma was a sensible girl. Wilma was my best friend. She did not abandon me after that spring, like so many others, when I took ill. Instead, she came more often, bringing books, crafts, pictures, magazines, ideas, giggles, etc.

Wilma was the most exquisite creature ever created. Almost mythical. In her presence, you sometimes felt as though you had been carted off to another dimension where these magical creatures reigned with an intelligence and tranquility unequaled in this realm. In her world lived only gods and goddesses, self-existent and immortal. They ruled over us mere mortals with a gentle, fervent ardor. I had never before, and have not since, laid eyes on anything quite so beautiful. Her skin was a conglomerate mixture of muted earth tones - creamy white with flakes of brown and orange and ochre spotted generously about. Her face was basically a flat, smooth surface, like a canvas with blobs of paint waiting to be smeared into order or disorder. The plane of her forehead emerged from her velvety hairline and turned almost immediately into flat, oval cheeks, devoid of cheekbone prominence, contoured into an indistinct chin. Her mouth was the most fetching of all. When she smiled, that mouth of hers would twist up onto one side of her face, leaving the other side mouthless. Needless to say, Wilma tried not to smile, but this was difficult for her because she was the silliest girl I have ever known.

For a few years when she was young, Wilma felt compelled to explain to everyone within audible range, that the surgeon, while operating on her ears in infancy, had severed a nerve, leaving her with that remarkable, most gratifying, crooked smile, although these were not her words, not exactly. Her nose was petite, not pointed, not quite flat; nevertheless, almost indistinguishable from the rest of her face. Her placid brown eyes had been positioned, demure and staid, under her eyebrows as though they were just a couple of brown buttons sewn on. She usually wore her long mousy-brown hair in two braids that hung right down to her bottom. Sometimes she tied them together with colored ribbons. She was thin and on the short side, and wore platform shoes and long skirts or wide legged jeans like the rest of us. We often traded clothing and wished we had been born sisters. We pricked our fingers, drew blood, pressed our bleeding fingers together, became blood sisters, swore to love one another for eternity.

I have kept that promise through all these years. Although it has been a silent covenant for a very long time now, it is not untouched for I often retrieve it from its cubby to remind myself that integrity in human form, within and without, does exist. Plus, I just like to think of Wilma and her smile.

Wilma. Oh Wilma....

Wilma's family moved to these Southern Alberta prairies from an Amish community in Pennsylvania. She had three sisters and three brothers. Wilma was third from the top, the eldest of the sisters. I saw her mother's hair undone once. It flowed over her shoulders, sweeping in long waves down her back right down to her knees, dusky black with defining streaks of silver, like a great glossy mane. It didn't seem to suit the rest of her pudgy body, which looked more like the Pillsbury doughboy than the figure of a mature woman. She was beautiful too, though her features were more normal than her eldest daughter's, and quite lovely. When she spoke to us, she used the pronoun *you*, or its plural, *yous*.

Do yous want some milk and woopy pies? Or, *Will yous be back for dinner?* Or sometimes, *Yous are just too silly today. Get out of here yous girls before I take the broom to your bottoms.*

Her eyes were bright and soft, her countenance kindly.

I thought that Wilma's mother lived her entire life in the kitchen. I see now, that this was an ignorantly absurd notion. She must have had a life elsewhere. For instance, she must have gone to the bathroom once in awhile. She must have dusted the living room on her journey from the kitchen, through the wide, cluttered hall, up the stairs and into the bedroom where all those freckled children must have been conceived. She must have had time to conceive them.

There was also a sewing room tucked tightly between all those crowded bedrooms. Spread out on the sewing table, and under the sewing machine's needle, an unfinished segment of some garment, quilt, or tablecloth, lay awaiting her masterful touch. She must have begun those projects and finished them outside the domain of her kitchen. She must have gone outside occasionally, for in the summer, immaculate rows of petunias and marigolds lined the walk. In the winter, eighteen boots in perfect military array, lined the porch floorboards and nine parkas hung from brass-coated hooks on the wall. Someone would have tidied them and I am certain it would not have been the handiwork of the children, except possibly for Wilma, who was perfect.

There was a sort of smelly comfort in that Amish household. Smelly, because of a diminished water supply, which necessitated that the toilet be flushed only after a b.m. Comforting, because it just was. I never really thought about that feeling of comfort and ease until now. It was just there, an all pervasive, but non-intrusive, entity.

Years later, when Wilma graduated from the University of Calgary with a Bachelor of Nursing degree, her parents and younger sisters threw her a party. There had to have been at least a hundred people there, all milling about the yard; in the vestibule, no longer lined with eighteen boots and nine parkas; in the living room, someone playing the piano, another tooting on an ancient recorder; upstairs, sprawled on the old bunks; hanging out the windows; some in the barn on stacks of square bales; some in the corral, stroking horses manes. Everybody loved Wilma. When I peeked into the house, Wilma's mother was bending over the hot stove, her long silver mane pulled up into a bun, a few strands near her temples moist with perspiration. She had oven mitts on and was taking out another tray of woopy pies.

Would yous like some iced tea with your woopy pies? she asked me.

Wilma said this to me,

Do you ever feel sometimes that you're the only important person in the world? That you're in the center and the rest of the world is just there because you're in the middle of it?

I didn't reply right away. We were only twelve years old and lying in the back of my parents' eggshell station wagon waiting for my mother to collect the groceries from the TomBoy Food Store. If my friend Wilma was the center of the universe, then maybe I was off just a little. Or maybe it was just us two. Maybe Wilma had her own universe to be the center of. The thing is, when Wilma said that to me, I didn't feel quite so alone anymore. I had a comrade. She never knew this about me. I never told her that I, too, felt stuck right in the middle, while everything else revolved, non-stop, around me. It made me dizzy sometimes, my eyes following the movements of that diffusive world. But it never slowed down enough for me to step off.

No, not really, I said.

Now I see that this is how we all should feel. We have to. It is our only means of defense against an antagonizing world of depersonalizing angst. We are told that in order to flourish in a productive, healthy manner, we must realize and acknowledge our own specialness, our uniqueness, that there is a separate path for every individual. We must become separate from our parents, our community of friends, relations. We must individuate in order to grow and eventually become an integral part of the collective whole. I find this to be a somewhat paradoxical notion. First, we are taught to detach, to

27

become undivided, complete beings on our own, able to function as an island before we can be of any useful benefit to the mainland. This is, of course, a uniquely western idea. Children of Asian and Eastern countries are socialized to integrate into the collective whole from the moment of birth. There is no recognizable individual, only families, groups of employees, communities, etc.

So here, in the Western Hemisphere anyhow, is the crux: to retain indivisibility, a kind of blending or dissolving, like salt in water, is to sustain a pathological deficiency. You are a failure. You have never grown up, never individuated. You are just a blobby mess, an egg without a shell. You might say that my desire for anonymity is a dysfunction, something that needs to be worked out. To reach full maturity I need to accept my individuality. Accept my limited parameters. Accept that I am unlike any other human being. Accept the whisperings, the criticisms, the sneers from other, more mature individuals, who have reached higher levels of actualization.

Yes, I am being cynical. Why not? I mean who's listening?

shshshshshshshshshshsh

Really, I must give myself a kick in the behind. Yesterday my husband was worrying about the cattle. He hadn't checked the fence line in over three weeks.

Tomorrow, he told me. *I'll try to get home a little early from work. I heard there was a wolf around, and I haven't counted those babies. It'd be terrible if we lost even one of them.*

It isn't fair, my husband having to work at the gas plant every day and come home to more work. I try with all my might, to get things done, so that he doesn't have to carry such a cumbersome load of physical responsibilities.

It's okay, I'll do it, is what I reply. And I will. Sometimes it's just a matter of mental determination, but I will get it done.

So I scrape myself up off my bed where I have been lying all this time after that last headstand. My head swims for a few moments. I close my eyes, breathe, count to six. I pull my socks on, straining. My back has seized up again. I roll my head, side to side, backwards, forwards, cracking out the kinks. A little bit of nausea throws me off kilter, then settles. I'm alright. I'm okay.

It is a beautiful late October day, supposed to reach a high of 16C by mid afternoon. I should be outside today anyway. I can't afford not to appreciate these wonderful gifts, and gifts they are. Soon there will be snowdrifts covering the driveway, the verandah, the windows. Getting dressed just to go outside will require insurmountable gusts of strength, pulling on extra wool socks, climbing into my snowsuit, trying to bend over to pull on my boots, then snugging the snowsuit leg around my boots to keep out the snow, shuffling through the mitt box for a pair of matching mittens, scarf, toque. By the time I am dressed I am so worn out that I have to sit down until breath returns. So I must take full advantage of these warm, quiescent, diminishing days of autumn.

I dress warmly, nevertheless. I can't afford to be chilled in the least. A slight drop in temperature and my body begins the hypothermia process. It begins to tense up, to conserve its meager resources, protect itself from the elements. With tension, there is pain. With pain there is more tension until my whole body is throbbing with agonizing pangs. So even though the sun is bright, the air warm, with barely a breeze to cast a chill, I tug on my thermal underwear, loose-fitting jeans, a sweatshirt, sweater and one of my husband's big red and black lumber jackets so that I will be able to maneuver myself inside all these heavy layers. I grab a knitted scarf from the mitt box, some mismatched gloves, lace up my boots and I'm set to go.

The leaves have almost all gravitated towards the ground now. I'm walking on a soft bed of damp leaves, twigs, mulch and loose earth. The landscape is a canvas of soft browns, muted orange, yellow and ashen gray. It looks and feels like Wilma's skin. The air is so still that I feel as though I am disrupting some sacred moment, those precious, hushed moments in which the earth grows sleepy and, inevitably, falls asleep.

I would like to go by horseback, but dare not risk the pain and discomfort it would, invariably, induce. Also, it is difficult for me to lift the saddle or raise my arms above my head to affix the bridle. My doctor advises that I must not, under any circumstance, attempt to raise my arms above my head or I will bring on another crash that could last for days. So Instead I will start up the quad. It will be a noisy and bumpy ride, its exhaust somewhat more toxic than what the horse would produce, but the quad will be quicker and more efficient. Later, I will spend time with the horses, stroking their scraggly manes, pressing my face against their long necks, breathing in that musky, oily aroma. I will feel comforted by that smell, gather strength from their hardiness, their taut, toned muscles. I will feel loved, protected, reassured, not quite so solitary. I indulge in these luxuries as often as I can.

Wilma and I used to ride. On a warm day nothing could surpass the absolute freedom of galloping over those endless patchwork prairies. Once we had memorized where the fence lines began and ended, or where a portion of fence was down, we could run, virtually unencumbered, over those vast golden prairie waves, our hair flying out behind us, the wind and bugs bringing tears to our eyes, laughing, unable to speak for breathlessness and sheer happiness. Sometimes we rode bareback and so that we could talk and giggle as girls do.

Wilma was a conscientious girl. I had recovered from my bout of the flu, or so we thought, but she was still protective, concerned for my well being, as I was for hers. I had returned to school with all of my school work completed, feeling somewhat abashed my first day back, still overly conscious about my collapsing stunt the previous week. But with renewed strength, my emotional state was also in check and I was determined to be more aware of my physical condition even if it meant asking permission to go to the bathroom or the water fountain. She stuck close to me those first few days. The fact, too, that she was my best friend, therefore allowed to glue herself to my side, was an enviable position to those who were admiring my ability to just fall out of my chair one day, thus prompting a week at home.

The whole class had signed a get-well card, even Stinky and the President. Somehow my illness had earned me some fame. Many of the girls were pressing Wilma for information, for permission to sit beside me. They wanted to touch me like they thought I was Jesus. But Wilma was not easily persuaded. If she felt so inclined, she would allow one or two questions to which she would respond only if she thought it a worthy inquiry.

I don't think she's up to it right now, she might say. Or, *I just don't think she feels much like talking. She's had a very long day.* Or, *Leave her alone for awhile. All this attention might make her faint again. She'll talk to you tomorrow.* And, *stop pushing!*

April had come around again. Our front lawn was immersed in a tepid, murky lake but some of the higher areas were almost dry and beginning to sprout alfalfa, grass, clover, and an assortment of other abundant prairie foliage. It was a Saturday I remember. Wilma had stayed the night upstairs in my attic room with the slanted ceiling, the two of us tucked into my single bed, chattering half the night away, and slumbering until well after ten o'clock the next morning. She braided my hair, which, when braided, barely touched my shoulders, not like her long roping braids that ended in ribbons just beyond the small of her back.

Around noon, we led my horse, Saber, into the barn, brushed him down, one of us on each side, caressing his neck and mane. I usually sat in front when we rode bareback because my legs were longer so that I could grip Saber with my knees if I had to, Wilma, behind me, clutching my waist, relying on my grip.

We rode past the house, followed the railroad tracks for awhile, then cut off going northward and uphill, into a small patch of shrubs and stunted spruce trees. This is all I remember. The rest I learned from my best friend later, after we had walked the two miles home and she was explaining to my frantic mother why we were covered in mud, scratched up as though we'd been in a fight with a lynx, and why Saber, less two riders, had beat us home.

I don't really know what happened. Saber started running. Not fast, but he was running. I think he was trying for a running jump over the ditch and onto the road.

Sometimes we do that. She just kind of slumped over - I was behind, holding on. So I held on tighter and hollered at her but she didn't say or do anything. Then she started falling over and I was afraid we'd both fall off. She said she felt funny, and then Saber took a leap. I grabbed the reins, but we both slid off and she was on the bottom. I think I fell right on top of her. I didn't mean to. I was just trying to keep us both on, but I forgot about that ditch. I got up right away, but Saber was already on the other side of the field by the time I figured out what had happened. Then she kind of moaned. I think she must have fainted again - before we fell off. I think that's what happened. I'm really sorry.

My mother's arms were around Wilma's shoulders. Wilma was crying, distraught, her words broken with sobs, those brown spots of eyes brimming and glassy with salty tears that dribbled into her crooked mouth while she spoke.

It's all right, Wilma. You're home now. You both got home. That's what's important. You're both here now and nobody's hurt. I should've known better than to let her go out so soon after being sick. Now don't you worry, you're both okay and that's all that's important. We'll just go in and warm up some soup and donuts, see?

But her arm. We're not okay. She's hurt her arm.

I realized then that I was clutching my left arm, cradling it in my right hand. We had tramped two miles across the prairies, climbed through barbed-wire fences, trudged up long, slow inclines, through coulees and spring sludge. We were muddy and wet, both of us crying, our egos bruised, our bodies throbbing from the fall. It felt like an elephant was standing on my arm. It wouldn't move. It just hung, limp, from my shoulder, braced against my body by my other arm.

Wilma's mother was called. Her father rambled up in their two-tone green station wagon. He was an uncomplicated man of many nervous smiles and very few words. I could hear the exchange between him and my mother at the door, my mother providing him with an explanation in her almost dreadfully detailed manner. Now and then I could hear a timid

33

half laugh and, *okay then,* or, *all right then,* at least half a dozen times; then two car doors slamming simultaneously and the sound of the family station wagon rumbling off down the driveway.

I spent a fitful night alone in my attic room. I had to lie absolutely still, or intense, biting pains knifed through my arm and shoulder till I felt nauseated and dizzy. I dozed through a series of catnaps, in which my dreams were pervaded by wild horses running amuck over rocky cliffs, falling on one another, bones, blood and guts spreading out over entire mountains. From those dreams I passed into another in which I was being suffocated by the earth itself, my face pressed into the ground, held down by an invisible force, as though the air itself had solidified and was holding me, immobile, crushing me into my own grave. I would wake with a start, my arm throbbing with slow, unremitting pulses. Twice during the night my mother tiptoed into my room. Once, I was awake but was too clouded in my own suffering to acknowledge her presence. I must have been partially asleep the second time for I could feel the soft coolness of her fingers stroking through my hair but could not shake myself awake. I wanted her to stay with me, but also wanted to be alone for I felt crowded, boxed in on all sides.

Wilma called the next morning, a Sunday as I recall, two short rings, one long, and although I was out of bed, propped up on the couch with a pillow to support my arm, I felt no inclination to speak with anyone, not even my best friend. I could hear my mother doing dishes in the kitchen, and could envision the phone cradled between her ear and shoulder as she again recited the whole, uncensored narrative to Wilma's mother, who, I am sure, was feeling somewhat responsible for the mishap.

Nine a.m. Monday morning found my mother and me bicycling the scant mile into town.

For heaven's sake, she scolded herself for weeks afterwards, and to anyone who happened to inquire about the sling encasing my arm. *Whatever could I have been thinking, making my daughter ride a bicycle into town that morning?*

34

Why, anything could have happened! And to think of that X-ray, well I just shudder to think of it, that bone broken right through and just hanging there. It looked like something you'd see in a horror picture. And no one in my family has ever had a broken bone. I just couldn't have guessed! And to think of those girls walking all that way home after the fall, too. Why, there had to have been a half-a-dozen fences to climb through. And I didn't even give her any aspirin. Oh whatever was I thinking!

First she took me to a friend of hers who was a nurse, although not practicing at the time. She asked me to remove my blouse so that she could view both shoulders at the same time to see if there was any variance between the two, any swelling, any sagging, any bulges or bruises where there shouldn't have been. I was mortified, of course, baring my undeveloped chest to a total stranger and was aghast that my mother would subject me to such embarrassment. But I complied silently as I usually did, not wanting to make any kind of fuss. She asked me to raise my right arm, which I did, then my left arm, which I couldn't do.

Does it hurt to raise your arm like that, or does it feel stuck and just won't go any further? she asked me.

Well both I think. It feels stuck because it hurts.

It's hard to say, she said, turning to my mother. *Maybe you should take her over to the infirmary, although I think it would be wise to have it X-rayed over at the hospital. You can't be too cautious about this kind of thing, especially in that area. It could be her shoulder. She could have dislocated it, but she's not very big so it's hard to tell.*

The two of them stood there gawking at my bare chest, discussing what should be done with me, as though I were only a configuration against a backdrop of kitchen counters and cupboards, and a sink full of dirty dishes.

Well, get dressed then, Honey.

She handed me my blouse and I turned around to put it on in an effort to reclaim a little bit of stolen dignity. The tea kettle whistled; boiling water was poured into a china tea pot

35

and set to steep for a few minutes while china cups and saucers were set upon a floral table cloth; toast crumbs were whisked away; shortbread cookies were fetched from the pantry and placed in a ring on a china plate which was then set in the center of the floral tablecloth; a glass bottle of fresh milk was retrieved from the porch, having been delivered earlier that morning, poured into a china cream pitcher and placed beside a china sugar bowl. It was a lovely tea, really, but for many days afterwards, my mother was unable to forgive herself for taking so much time to get to the hospital.

For heaven's sake, she would declare with a shake of her strawberry blonde head, *how could I have done that, first bicycling all the way into town, making her stand there like that when she was hurting so much, then having tea, then going to the infirmary? Why couldn't I have just driven her to the hospital in the beginning? Oh, what was I thinking anyway? Heavens! Sometimes I just don't know!*

After the lovely tea with the nurse, we peddled towards the school infirmary, my mother slightly ahead of me, her panty-hose clad legs sticking out beneath a knee-length floral print dress that could have been made from the same material as the nurse's table cloth; and me, a few peddles behind, clutching the handlebar with my good arm, hugging the other close to my chest.

Thankfully, the nurse in the infirmary did not insist I take off my shirt to be examined. In fact, she did not even touch me. She merely asked if I could raise my arm, which I couldn't, so off we peddled five more blocks to the hospital this time.

My mother sat there on a bench in the radiology waiting area while I was ushered into the darkened X-ray room. After fifteen minutes or so, the doctor opened the door and asked her to join us. I was proudly gazing at the spectacular photo of my broken bone when she walked in. I heard a distinct gasp while the doctor quickly shoved a chair underneath her as she slumped into it.

Oh! Oh my! What is that? Oh, dear, oh, heavens! she

cried, her hands slapped across her cheeks, a dumbfounded look of shock and disbelief in her eyes. *Oh, my! What have I done? Is that - is that a bone? Her bone? Is that - oh, no, it couldn't be, it just couldn't! Oh, Honey, what did you do? Is it broken?*

The doctor merely chuckled.

Well, yes, that is an X-ray of your daughter's arm, he said pointing to the injury, tapping the screen with his index finger. *You can see it's just a small fracture. Children heal quickly. Their bones are still growing, still pliable.* But my mother was horrified, almost dumbstruck for once. Her hands slid down her pallid face, where they clasped each other in her lap. She was visibly shaking.

Will she - will she have to wear a cast?

I was very excited. It wasn't hurting nearly as much now. The pain had spread up through my shoulder, but it was dull, bearable. I looked again at the X-ray, at the jagged edges of the fracture, which looked like the jaws of a shark ready to clench down on its prey and tear it to bloody bits. I wanted to take that picture home with me, frame it, hang it on my bedroom wall, color it a little, give it some life. Honor it like some sort of credential, a diploma, like those I'd seen on the wall of the doctor's office.

I don't think so. Really, I think it would just be an unnecessary discomfort. Up there so close to the shoulder, it would be hard to fit, unless we put a sort of body cast right around both shoulders. No, I think we'll just fit her with a sling. She'll have to keep it immobile - completely still - in order for it to heal properly though. Can you deal with that? is what he asked me while I was busy being sorely disappointed that I wasn't going to get a cast after-all. I nodded. But my mother had recovered her tongue again.

She fell off her horse, you know. Did she tell you that?

Yes, she did. It happens. You're lucky it wasn't worse. Is the horse okay? he joked, attempting to lighten the mood for my mother's sake. But she wasn't easily distracted.

Did she tell you why she fell off her horse? She fainted,

that's why. She fainted and then fell off. Her friend fell on top of her, then they walked two miles home, through fences and mud and everything. She fainted and that's why she fell off her horse. She hasn't been feeling well, you know. Just a week ago, she fainted dead away right in school and I had to go pick her up. That's not normal, is it, to faint twice in one week?

Well, no, not usually. She could be a little anemic. How is her menstrual cycle?

At this, I cringed inwardly, my cheeks flushed. It was turning out to be another splendid day for humiliation. First I'd had to take my shirt off and pose for a stranger, now another stranger was prying into some very private matters, the kind of matters you only discussed with your very best friend, and then only in utter secrecy. My mother looked over expectantly at me and for a brief moment, although it seemed like an eternity, no one spoke.

Well? urged my mother.

I don't - I haven't – I stammered.

I don't think she's begun that yet, Doctor. But she hasn't been eating much either. She's been a little tired.

Well why don't you bring her over to the clinic tomorrow and we'll just run a couple of tests just to rule things out. It can't hurt. A girl her age shouldn't be tired and fainting all the time. More than likely it is hormonal.

He called in a nurse who brought with her a square of light canvas cloth and a large safety pin. She placed my left hand across the right side of my chest so that my fingers touched my neck; folded that square cloth into a triangle; tucked it beneath the injured arm; wrapped it around my neck and tied it into a bulky knot that pinched the skin on the back of my neck; and then tucked up the loose end around my elbow, securing it with the safety pin.

There you go now, smiled the nurse. *You should wear it all the time if possible, even at night.*

Well now, what are we to do? We've ridden our bicycles into town. You can't ride a bike with a broken arm, said my mother as we walked briskly back down the wide hospital corridor. She seemed to have forgotten that we'd just ridden about two miles already that morning and were no worse off for it.

We'll have to call your father to come and get us. Oh, will he be surprised! My goodness!. Oh, I just can't get that image out of my mind, that broken bone. I've never seen anything like it. Oh, it makes me shudder to think of it. I should have known better than to have you and that horse running about all over the country when you'd been sick. Well, never mind that now. I'll see to it that it heals properly. Maybe we should make a bed for you downstairs. I don't know that you should be running up and down those stairs. Oh, what if you fainted again and fell? Oh, and what about the bus? I will telephone the bus driver and have her reserve the front seat for you. I can just see you getting jostled about and hurting that arm again.

She stopped at the front phone booth, fished in her purse for a dime, dialed the number and then I could see her lips moving rapidly again, that worried look upon her face. Within minutes, my father rumbled up to the emergency entrance.

I smiled when he tapped my broken arm, but my mother quickly nudged him away.

Oh no, Father. She is to keep it absolutely still or it won't heal. Can you believe it? She's broken her arm. The first broken bone in my family. Why, you should have seen the X-ray. It was like something out of a horror picture. I just couldn't believe it, and me, making her ride her bicycle all the way into town this morning. Sometimes I just really wonder about myself. What kind of mother am I anyway?

My father smiled at me, tapping my arm again.

No cast? What kind of broken bone can you have with no cast? How is anybody to sign a sling? Well I will be the first.

And he drew out of his breast pocket, a black, felt-tipped pen, with which he proceeded to draw a stick figure with a jagged-edged arm protruding awkwardly from its stick chest and wrote, *I love you, Father.* Only Wilma was allowed to draw another picture on my sling. No one else.

It's just a bone, Mother. It will heal. It's still intact. It hasn't fallen off. It could have been much worse. He opened up the back of our station wagon and managed to cram both of our bicycles inside.

So you rode your bike into town with a broken arm eh? he chuckled.

I slid into the front center while my mother and father took their respective positions. My mother kept shaking her head. My father was whistling, pleased with the unexpected opportunity to be called away from work. I knew he would take the rest of the day off, tell his supervisor that his daughter had been injured and had to be taken to the hospital, even if the injury had taken place days before. He would sit in his chair by the fireplace and read the paper until supper, after which he would, no doubt, plunk himself back into the chair again and fall asleep.

I loved my parents deeply, even then, at an age when most children were indifferent to their parents. My father, the lovable, forgetful, and sometimes mindless man, was never in a hurry, never quick to speak or judge, could always fit one more mouthful of stew into his mouth, and always had time for me, his one and only child. There was more security and comfort in that household than a child would need in a lifetime. So why did I feel neglected and afraid?

Wilma's mother drove her over after supper and stayed while Wilma and I chattered in excited, hushed tones in the living room, my father snoring blissfully in his chair. I could hear my mother in the kitchen repeating, in minute detail, all that had transpired during the past twelve hours, and Wilma's patient mother, interjecting quick, dutiful apologies.

I told them. I said, Yous girls be careful now. Them fields are soft and slippery sometimes in the spring. Wilma's feeling very badly. But I told her. I said, Yous girls just get too silly sometimes. Why can't yous just stay in the house or in the yard? is what I said to her.

Next morning, my mother was flipping through a Canadian Circle magazine, perched, straight-backed and solemn, on a wooden chair in the doctor's office waiting room. I sat beside her, sleepy, and clutching my arm after another fitful night.

Thus began a year of unavailing blood tests, peeing in plastic cups, being poked and thumped and assessed by all kinds of doctors, in all kinds of clinics, some so shoddy and smelly you were afraid to breath for fear of catching something terminal, and some so modern and stilted you were afraid to breath for fear of offending someone.

shshshshshshshshshshsh

The first couple of visits were extensive and somewhat wearying, packed with questions, laboratory requisitions, needles, which I didn't mind so much, and further X-rays, most of it an unfamiliarity. My mother was adamant that I be checked over with grueling thoroughness. The first doctor, who had been responsible for that marvelous photo of my broken limb, suggested that I be assessed for mononucleosis as he told us that a few local cases had surfaced over the past year. So for the next few days, with every opportunity my mother could conjure up, she was informing everyone that her daughter had mono.

The doctor says its most likely mono. Now, tell me, where would she have picked up something like that? Nobody in my family has ever been sick with anything for more than a day. She'll be in bed for months, is what I've heard about mono. I've got to get her on some vitamins, that's what. Vitamin B complex, iron. I know what I'll do. I'll run over to the health food store and pick up some brewer's yeast. I've heard it cures just about anything if you can get it down.

Mono, eh? said my mirthful father in a pensive tone, his thumb and index finger tapping his whiskered chin. *Isn't that the kissing disease? Now who have you been kissing, eh?*

Just you, Father, I returned.

Well one thing's for sure, you haven't lost the wit you inherited from your father. You'll be okay. Don't you worry.

He patted my injured arm again much to the dismay of

42

my mother who had not gotten her way about setting up a bed for me in the living room. She did, however, manage to talk the bus driver into saving the entire front seat for me which, to me, was just one more advertisement regarding my physical state than I wanted. I was, however, quickly growing accustomed to the attention. But after a month of missing school, arriving late, or leaving early, I was relieved to have nearly lost my novelty status amongst my classmates.

It wasn't mono. My mother seemed almost disappointed and tried to enlist my father's support in insisting that the doctor administer the blood test a second time.

There's really no point, he said from behind his daily newspaper. *I'm sure the doc knows what he's doing. And anyway, shouldn't we be thankful that she doesn't have mono? He said it's probably some sort of virus, right? Nothing to worry about. Isn't that right, Baby Doll?* he said to me, his soft, laughing eyes peering out from above his paper.

I do feel better, is what I said with all the assurance I could muster up. *I mean I don't feel quite so dizzy and my arm doesn't hurt much at all.* And then a little louder so that my mother could hear from her semi-permanent stance at the kitchen sink, *I think it's healed enough for me to sit in my regular seat on the bus, even.*

We're not even going to take a chance on that, Honey, is what I heard from above the clatter of pots and pans. *He said six weeks. It's only been four.*

My father winked at me. *Better listen to the boss, eh? After-all, she didn't arrive at that position for being a dilly, you know. Your mother does know best.*

What my mother didn't know was that the sling came off at night. I had difficulty enough getting to sleep those nights even without it, and still my nights were often pervaded with perturbing dreams, rolling one into another like a train car pile-up. Sometimes I would flick on the lamp during the night after a particularly troublesome dream. Some nights I left the light shining just to keep the darkness from invading my sleep and dreams. By ten o'clock most mornings, the grogginess would be tugging at me from every possible angle. My head would feel like a basketball filled with cement and my limbs would threaten to fall right off if I insisted that they carry me through the day.

It wasn't long after the horse incident that getting to school in the morning was out of the question. Instead, my mother insisted I sleep in for as long as I could, which was a relief since I seemed only to sleep during those morning hours anyway, after the darkness had melted away.

One evening in early May my father rumbled into the driveway, parking a little more delicately than his usual almost-sideswiping-the-garage manner. I peered out of the kitchen window, watching with curiosity as he jumped out of the driver's side and hopped around to the passenger side to open the door for a very tall, very odd looking woman, who pulled out of the car with her, a large tote bag and an overcoat draped over her arm. She smoothed her skirt, adjusted her horn-rimmed glasses, mouthed a brisk *thank you* to my father, who nodded and smiled in acknowledgment, and from the looks of things, made some well-meaning, comical remark to which that lofty woman did not respond other than a half smile which could have been interpreted as a grimace.

Who's she? is what I whispered to my mother who was also observing the scene from behind the safety of the kitchen window.

Oh, that must be your new tutor. Your father hired her to help you with some of your schoolwork so that you wouldn't get too far behind, missing all this school. I believe she's Dutch, from Holland I think, and has a funny accent. She says her ths like ds, but you must pretend you don't notice. She teaches school over in Trochu, grade five, I think.

Well she looks very scary.

Yes, I guess she kind of does, doesn't she, my mother commented in a low voice, shielding her mouth with her hand as though they might have heard us her through two window panes and halfway across the yard. *But you be nice to her*

44

anyway. She's going way out of her way to come here once a week, and you best show her your appreciation.

And she was, indeed, a very scary woman. She had to have been at least six feet tall, wore a pleated woolen skirt, a short-sleeved cashmere sweater, thick beige leotards and white running shoes, an odd combination I thought. But what did I know of Dutch people? I always thought they wore wooden shoes and aprons. Her short, plain brown hair was bound in curls so tight and stiff you probably could have bounced a rubber ball off of it. She smelled faintly of Lysol and lanolin. Her hands were a labyrinth of lines and veins; long, thin, crooked fingers, bony knuckles, and flat fingernails cut so short I could see the red rim where a normal fingernail would still be in place even trimmed right down to the end of the finger. With these skeletal hands, she unlatched her tote bag, drew out some familiar textbooks, set them on the table, and without waiting for an introduction, sat herself down, motioned for me to follow suit, and thus, I was initiated into my first student-tutor session.

She was certainly an adept teacher and tutor. She was thorough and exhibited neither patience nor impatience with me, but merely explained each situation once, twice, or thrice, which was usually more than sufficient. It appeared she had no sense of humor whatsoever, for each of my father's attempts at joviality was simply disregarded as irrelevant and unnecessary.

Each Thursday, this strange monolith of a lady appeared at our door, chauffeured from Trochu by my father and back to town an hour and a half hence, not a moment later.

I supposed she had never married because I could not fathom what man would want her for a wife, although no personal information was ever offered to us at all. I also assumed she had no family or close friends because she always wore the same drab, lifeless clothing, and usually it was up to one's friends to remind one of the appropriate fashions. I couldn't even imagine what sort of underthings she might wear and quite frankly, considering her without clothing was a rather frightening concept so I pushed it out of my mind. I had not

45

seen jeweled, horn-rimmed glasses on anyone else except in very old class photos lining the school hallway walls. Apparently, this woman was an anachronism, so I decided, rather than turn up my nose at her archaic style, to utilize the opportunity to glimpse into this very precise, obsolete, world into which she had captured herself. I decided to amuse myself with her large uncomely hands, turning them into the crafty hands of a black sorceress. I adorned her with dark, fur-lined robes and crowned her with gaudy jewels; I gave her long wisps of crimson hair that trailed on the ground behind her and wound around her austere countenance like rivulets of blood; her voice became larger and more ominous; that faint whiff of Lysol and lanolin became the damp, despairing smell of her prisoners' cells; and her pencil became a wand with which she would, on a whim and a cackle, turn people into stone.

But all these wondrous fantasies that I projected onto my tutor were quickly dispelled, when on the third session she brought with her a small tin box with a hinged lid.

I brought these for you, is what she said placing the box on the table before me, and then commanded, *go ahead, open it up*. And so I did. Inside was a double layer of flat, black squares, which emitted a potent licorice scent. *I brought you some Dutch licorice. Go ahead, try one. Not only is it very tasty, but is also good for an ailing tummy.*

Gingerly, I broke off one square from the slab inside the tin box and placed it on the end of my tongue, hoping that I wouldn't have to make a fool of myself or displease her by spitting it out or gagging on it. Instantly my saliva glands began to sweat profusely with the unfamiliar taste sensation. I rolled it around on my tongue, twisting it from side to side. It was not at all like the black licorice sticks we bought downtown at the TomBoy. It was stronger, less sweet and quite salty. There was a much sharper zing to it, unpretentious, bold.

Yum! is what I heard myself exclaim, breaking another square away and popping it into my watering mouth.

They're meant to be dissolved in the mouth, she

admonished. *You don't chew them up like regular candy. You're to savor the taste. Now put them away and let's get to our lesson.*

It was somewhat astonishing, at first, to perceive this towering, statuesque lady in mere human terms. But a funny thing happened. I began to see her almost eye to eye. One to one. I began to realize that although she was taller, older, possibly eccentric, and certainly more learned than I, we shared nearly the same space in this vast universe. There in the kitchen of my parents' aged farmhouse, that great lady and I became comrades of a sort. She never said as much, not aloud. But she liked me. I know she did. Each week a new tin container of Dutch licorice was set before me on the table. Each week I popped two pieces into my mouth immediately and set the rest aside for later in the week. I knew that it pleased her to see me devouring her treasures so readily but she never failed to exhort me in the practice of moderation. I may have been what many students coined, teacher's pet, but since these were private sessions, I was able to lap up all of her unspoken approval without the disapproval of my peers.

And this is how the spring passed. My arm healed quickly, but even after six weeks my mother would gasp involuntarily every time she heard me thundering down our spiral staircase, unintentionally slamming the front door, or rocking in our squeaky rocking chair.

It just makes me think of broken bones grinding together, like Ezekiel's valley of dry bones. That's all I can think of when I hear that sound, a heap of broken bones. It just makes me shudder, is what she said. *And what I don't want is to have to go look at another X-ray of another broken bone. That would be enough to send me right over the edge!*

What she didn't know was that Wilma and I had not slowed our rambunctiousness, not a single pace. Wilma's father was a dairyman. The dairy barn, where he worked from before sun up to well past sun down, and where Wilma and I spent the majority of our time together, was, to me, a castle of sorts, riddled with trap doors and tunnels and chutes that led one into another. We would spend entire afternoons trailing one another on our hands and knees through tunnels constructed from hundreds of hay bales. A single game of hide and seek might take hours within the myriad burrows, doors and piles of loose hay in which to conceal ourselves. By the end of a day, the two of us would be itching in the most unimaginable places, scratched raw from the rough wooden beams, and hurriedly yanking hay from our tousled hair before Wilma's mother could threaten to throw us both into the cream separator.

How I managed to fall from above the second floor through a bale chute onto the concrete floor below still evades my conscious memory. But there I was, kneeling on that cold cement floor in the midst of a dozen cows' rumps and their milking machines, the sweet-sour odor of manure and warm milk, and the vibrating timbre of cows mooing amongst themselves.

It took Wilma a little longer to find me that time. After she had searched the entire upper floor and its labyrinth of bales, she began calling my name. Wilma knew every hiding spot in that barn and it was just a matter of picking the right one. But this time it seemed I had disappeared, she told me later, absorbed right into the cobwebbed walls. After awhile she poked her head into the bale chute again just to be sure. Her eyes adjusting to the darkness, she scanned it from top to bottom and then noted that the floor board had come unlatched and was hanging down below into the milking arena. A second look brought into focus what appeared to be someone on the cement floor below, praying. She must have called to me then, but I don't recall hearing her voice, only the mooing and swishing of tails and pawing at the hay.

Moments later she was at my side with that funny smile of hers squished up onto the right side of her face.

What're you doing? is what she asked, breathless. I tried to think of what had just happened, but all I could remember was bracing myself against the four sides of that chute. I must have jumped or fallen down from my perch, the floor opened up, and gravity whizzed me right through to the concrete base below. When Wilma could elicit no response from me, she looked up at the board dangling by a rope near the ceiling.

Oh, is what she said. Then, *OOOH!* Her mouth returned to its position near the center of her face, her brown button eyes widened, scanning the scene again, up to the ceiling, down to the prayerful figure on the concrete.

Uh oh, she said. *You fell, didn't you. You fell through the feeding chute. Can you move?*

I drew in a deep, painful breath, the first since my arrival by air onto that incredibly hard floor. That breath made me topple right over onto my nose where I teetered for a precarious moment, then clunked over onto my side, my knees still tucked up to my belly.

I don't know. I don't think so. I think I'm dead. Am I dead, Wilma?

She shook her head, almost sadly, her long braids bobbing from side to side. Then her mouth began to twitch and quiver and all at once it shot up onto the side of her beautiful face again,

Great hiding place, huh? is what I breathed, my head rolling over onto the concrete, my legs stubbornly stretching out to their full length again. The cows were barely mindful of the intrusion, their great impassive faces turned towards us, peering over their massive rumps, munching, swishing, mooing, stomping, pawing.

Don't tell my mother, was the next thing that came to mind.

Well if you can get up and walk out of here, then we won't have to tell anybody. You're getting clumsy! She reached down and pulled me to my feet. I groaned. *You didn't faint again, did you?*

I didn't remember feeling faint at all, but my balance and depth perception had been misguiding me lately. Sometimes I would stumble over something that I thought was ten feet away, or I would miss a step on the stairway, causing my mother to wince again, clasping her hands over her heart.

Heavens! she would exclaim. *Have you got two left feet, Honey? Slow down! You're not competing in the hundred-yard dash you know.*

I stood, finding my breath again, a gripping tightness clenching my spine.

Are you sure you're okay? Wilma asked me. *You must have landed on your feet, I think. We better go latch up the chute though. You wait here. I'll run up and get it.* Wilma was a butterfly on her feet, so light and agile, never missing a step. Off she trotted to the back stairwell, skipping up two at a time. After a few moments I heard some shuffling above, and lifted my eyes to where I could see Wilma's speckled hands hauling up the floorboard by the rope and reattaching it. Then I could hear her quick footsteps pattering back across the upstairs floor and down the stairs. She grinned at me again.

You're really funny, is what she said, poking me in the ribs. *You shoulda seen yourself, looking all stunned and stupid. I guess I forgot about that board though. I shoulda told you, but now you know.*

Yeh, now I know. And I did feel stunned. My limbs were developing minds of their own, not heeding the commands my brain was trying to communicate to them. There seemed to be no synergy of movement, each of my components operating without regard for the other two thousand parts. Sometimes my hands and feet were so cold and stiff that I felt awkward trying to maneuver those appendages that seemed more like prophylactics than my own flesh.

Wilma walked me part way home via the railroad tracks, she, balancing perfectly on the metal rims, both arms stretched out on either side of her, and I, just trying to keep my balance stepping from tie to tie. We parted when the tracks veered northward and I headed east, about half a mile cross country, then through a gap in the caragana hedge and into the house through the back porch door.

It felt like my body had been compressed about six inches. There was a numbness settling through my spine, seeping down into my legs. I wondered how long I would be able to conceal my latest misadventure from my omniscient mother but needn't have wondered at all for the moment I walked in, she turned from the sink, grasped me by the shoulders, gathered in one of her all absorbing looks and gasped,

Lord in heaven what happened to you?

I stood mute before her, unable to attach words to the dull, stiff pain that was arching through my body and curious also, as to how my mother could instantly recognize that pain.

You're in shreds! Just look at you. You look like you've been in a lions' den! Whatever have you done this time? She tugged at my shirt sleeve which I then saw was torn from the shoulder to the elbow, and then she knelt on the floor and with her sudsy fingers, examined my pant legs, which I then realized were also torn out revealing a pair of badly bruised knee caps.

Lord have mercy, she sighed, shaking her head, *what will you think of next?*

Away we went to see another doctor again, this time in Red Deer, referred to us by my mother's nurse friend who had thoughtlessly asked me to bare all for her. He was old, this doctor, bald on top, with a few thin wisps of white hair scattered around his temples. He listened, a little impatiently I thought, to my mother's detailed account about how clumsy, weak, sleepy and achy I seemed to have become. He appeared to be particularly interested in the fact that most mornings I slept in, attended school only in the afternoons yet still had enough energy to fall out of barn lofts and off of horses.

Does she like school? is what he asked, flipping his pen from one side to the other.

Hasn't missed a day in her life until now.

How about friends then? Does she have many friends?

If she didn't have friends, she wouldn't be falling out of barns and such, my mother told him with a sudden air of impudence. *Yes, she has plenty of friends, good friends. Her whole class sent her a get well card.*

It was apparent that she had sensed where this line of

questioning was leading and was becoming impatient herself. She joined her hands in her lap, crossed her legs, her foot tapping impatiently against the bare floor.

If you are trying to suggest that my daughter is unhappy and is making all of this up - well you are wrong then. It isn't right that a twelve-year-old girl should be tired all the time no matter what the reason. But I tell you, my daughter is quite happy, other than her physical state. And I didn't drive all the way up here today to be told that it is in her head, or mine for that matter. If that's what you're going to say, then we shall just find ourselves a real doctor!

I hadn't known my mother was capable of displaying such open impetuosity and was taken aback at this sudden turn, feeling comforted and proud that my well- being was the forefront of her motivation.

All I'm saying, he continued, his high-pitched voice unwavering, *is that a thorough investigation must include all possibilities. I've seen this kind of thing before, the tiredness, the lack of appetite. There is a condition becoming prevalent in young girls, called anorexia nervosa. They literally starve themselves to death - but if you don't want to pursue it -*

My mother's face was reddening, her cheeks twitching, her lips tightening.

But, the doctor cleared his throat, tapping his pen on the table, aware of her mounting frustration, *there are a couple of other possibilities. She should be checked for Hepatitis and Meniere's disease, neither of which are very likely, but just to rule them out, all the same.*

She relaxed a little then, agreed to have the necessary tests and away we went again. That was the last doctor I saw for awhile. Instead, after the test results came back negative, my mother paid regular visits to the health food store down by the Bottle Depot. She bought me one of those pill organizers, a compartment for every day of the week, and filled it with every kind of vitamin and mineral imaginable, some of them grotesquely huge and unswallowable. She concocted brewer's yeast shakes in the blender and vegetable juices with her brand new juicer. She eliminated white sugar from my diet, then white flour. She curdled milk to make cottage cheese and then baked cottage cheese pizzas with whole wheat flour. She made blended spinach soup and attempted to disguise liver in a stew or ground it into a puree and spread between two slices of bread camouflaged under layers of tomatoes and lettuce. She grew alfalfa sprouts and bean sprouts in jars in the kitchen window, which my father and I consumed dutifully, like bunnies. For desserts we had home-canned fruit topped with homemade granola and fresh yogurt, or carob and honey brownies which tasted like sweetened cardboard.

Bless her indomitable soul, that mother of mine. What she didn't know was that I began hanging around in Wilma's mother's kitchen with her hot, sugary, chocolaty, woopy pies.

Now my mother feeds me brownies made from the whitest, most refined sugar money can buy.

If it's not going to make a difference in how you feel, then you may as well enjoy what you eat, is how she justifies herself plunking a hot pan of oven-fresh brownies in front of my watering mouth and undisciplined will-power. Still, I do have to watch what I eat. One of my mother's brownies could puff me up for an entire day, maybe two.

shshshshshshshshshshsh

The air is so fresh and crisp. I breath it in deeply, right down into my toes, remembering that any ailment should be curable simply by practicing proper breathing techniques and one must always be mindful of this. The air here is about as clear as it gets, despite toxic fumes from the highway less than half a mile away, the gas plants and oil wells, and, of course, cow farts. There are those fitness-obsessed people in the cities who run ten miles a day through city smog, which is far more toxic than cow farts, I should think.

I have come upon the first gate now. I gear down slowly so as to avoid the sudden lurches, which, if I'm not careful, can practically toss me head over heels. My husband has macgyvered the gate here with a rope instead of the usual barbed wire latch. This way I can let myself in and out easily without help. I untie the rope, slowly let out the slack until the wire is loose enough for me to lift the pole from the bottom rung and lower the gate to the ground. I hop back onto the quad and ease it over the prostrate gate, hop back off, lift the gate, thrust the pole back into place, wrap the rope around the fence pole, tighten it, tie it off, climb back onto the quad and follow the fence line for another quarter mile. It looks good. None of the bulls has tried to jump over and only a couple of small branches has broken off and fallen across the fence which I easily lift and toss onto the other side where I will pick them up later and throw them into a pile for burning this winter.

The cows have mangled the ground in places, which makes for a very bumpy ride. I try to remain loose, relaxed, but feel my back tightening anyway, my body's attempt to keep its inner organs from becoming all jumbled up. With one hand I steer, the other holds my breasts, which are quite sore today. Six years ago I had a hysterectomy which eliminated the severe pelvic pain twenty one days out of the month, but did nothing for other symptoms, the bloating and soreness surrounding my ovaries and the ten day swelling and lactation in my breasts every month. Today must be about day four. They are heavy and tender, beginning to leak. There have been days I've had to stuff tissues inside my bra to absorb the wetness. My husband massages them with his big, rough hands to ease the lumps. It hurts like all get out but afterwards they are less swollen and I can move about without so much discomfort.

In the distance I see a light cloudy mist suspended over the river valley. I have never been there. I have only sat in my rocking chair on the verandah, wrapped in a quilt, gazing out across this beautiful landscape, or as I'm doing now, atop four rugged tires and the sputtering rumble of the quad. It looks to be only about a mile, cross-country, where the hay fields meet bush and then descend to the riverbank. Beyond that the trees become hazy as they ascend once again into the splendor of an almost untouched wilderness.

This time of year, I used to like to imagine God, the ultimate artist, constantly adding to, never subtracting from, his ever-expanding canvas. Lately though, I have begun to eliminate God from having anything but a minuscule role in this wondrous composition. To consider God as a separate entity, the mastermind of this, and perhaps many other universes, tends to separate oneself from the circle, a circle in which there is no beginning and no end. A circle in which all things, living or not, are conjoined to fashion one unified essence which breathes in and out just as we do. The universe, I've read, is presently on an inward breath, expanding, creating, maturing. What happens when it reaches its full capacity and must begin to expel, to purge, collapse? Does it begin again? I don't think we are meant to wonder about such things but I can't help myself. I have too much time to think about these things that matter little in the speck of one's lifetime.

I will ponder, instead, on the way the river must look today. I will imagine the bubbling swirls of water rising and falling as they effortlessly maneuver themselves between and over pebbles and boulders. I will imagine the sound and swish of murmurs as the river gurgles and chatters, pursuing its course downstream, flowing, without thought, without effort. This is the Taoist concept of non-action and non-thought. To live as we ought is to live as the river flows. It just flows. It just is. It doesn't go anywhere in particular. It doesn't come from anywhere but itself. It just is.

I will imagine the cool dampness of the air hovering in the river valley. My skin will drink of it, absorbing it into my soul where it will purify and revitalize these heavy, tired thoughts I lug around with me. It will permeate every cell and bathe me in its cool, vital fertility. I will watch multi-hued leaves drift down from the trees, settling themselves on the river's ever-changing, wavering, mirrored surface. I will feel myself lift right off my weary feet and I will become Thumbelina and will alight onto one of these crisp, leafy boats and will allow myself to be carried along with the current wherever it shall take me. I shall have no thoughts, no pain. I shall just be.

Better than imagining, when I have completed this fence inspection, I will park the quad in the garage and I will put on my walking shoes. Today I will walk to the river, to that particular place at the edge of our property line where I have never been. I have often driven down to the campground along the highway, only about six miles from here, where I park in the last stall, lock up, then follow a game trail up-river to a secluded sandy arm where the river branches into a fork and joins again, encasing this tiny island in its own exclusive Eden.

I often remove my shoes first, hide them beneath the underbrush and skip barefoot from rock to rock, daring myself to maintain balance. Sometimes I do. Most times I do not, which is why I don't wear shoes.

Sometimes, once I have reached a safe distance from the campground, I remove all of my clothing, place them within reach on a dry rock, then ease myself down into the gritty, muddy sand. I smooth it over my entire body, first my toes and feet, then I work my way up my legs. It is cool and weighty, but not heavy, not like clothing. It is not a covering, but rather, it is nourishment. This is a ritual of sorts, perhaps much like the way the Natives smudge themselves for purification, to open eyes, ears and mouth to understanding and healing. Another fistful of mud is smoothed over my knobby knees, my thighs. I even smear it into the triangle of fuzzy hair between my legs, rub it over my bottom and the small of my back. Another scoop goes over my belly, filling the small dent of my navel. I must lift each teardrop breast to smooth it under them, and over, not too harshly for they are always so tender. The skin on my neck and shoulders is also very sensitive so I massage it in more gently, but my face can take a lot of grit. I even rub a bit in my ears and over my eyelids. What is left in my hands gets brushed through my hair.

I suppose one might also think of this as a baptism, covering myself with the earth then allowing the river to flow over my muddied body, carrying away impurities, enriching me with simplicity and clarity of vision. Nothing matters at this point. I know it will all wash off and if, perchance, anyone were to wander along at that moment, it wouldn't matter because I wouldn't see or hear them. The embarrassment would be theirs only, although I do not like to think of offending anyone and that has happened on more than one occasion. I have a knack for offending certain people with what seems to me, perfectly acceptable, natural behaviors. I must remember that it is the person who chooses to be offended. It is not my actions. I do try to keep my oddities to myself, but that is all I can control, not, for instance, a certain relation's response to those oddities.

This particular relative said this to me once;

It is abhorrent that you should expose your body, even if you think no one is watching. Why do you suppose God clothed Adam and Eve? They were naked, and ashamed. And what happened when the demons left the naked man and entered the herd of pigs? He clothed himself right away, that's what.

Under my breath I said, *and God forbid that we should all be born naked!* She didn't hear me say this of course because she was still yapping.

It's perversion, that's what it is, and you're only fooling yourself if you think it's not. And you wonder why we won't allow our children over here? Would you? I mean, really, think about it. With what goes on around here, I would be afraid to let my dog loose, a female dog at that!

Bitch, I think, is the correct term, is how I responded while her lips were still flapping like plastic in the wind.

Well! she huffed, *you are really troubled! You need help. Do you think we don't know? Do you really think you're hiding anything? People can tell just by the way you look. Nobody trusts you with their kids. And we also know what kind of people you've got consorting here - that gay friend of yours bringing all his homosexual friends around. Well I don't even want to know!*

It is true. I do have a gay friend. We met at an Esso station in Red Deer. He is the kindest, most considerate, non-judging person I know, next to Wilma. My gay friend, who lives too far away from me, would never even consider slandering another person like this. He also believes in treating all of God's creatures with dignity and respect. I could wax religious and say that my gay friend is the most Christ-like person I know, even more so than Wilma. Wilma did have a bit of a mean streak, which only made her more beautiful but also brought her back into the realm of Ordinary.

Nevertheless I was all torn up when these words were heaved at me, a spear intended to pierce my sensitive spirit, and it did. It pierced. But not the way she intended. I felt sad that someone would attempt to stomp on my means of worship. Other people may dress in their finest, go to church, plop themselves in pews, gripping hymnals in one hand, a Bible in the other. They might sing and pray loud enough to be heard in the church across town. I don't denigrate their forms of worship. It is their way of meeting their God. My manner of reverence is to remove all barriers and go to Him, or Her, or It, empty and naked so that I may be purged and filled. I'm afraid I don't quite understand the motivation behind their punitive sort of judgment. There are a lot of things I don't understand. I also know that I could be wrong. But it just doesn't feel very wrong. I think I would know, wouldn't I?

But again, this is alright with me. It has to be. I cannot defend myself. I wouldn't want to. I have no need of defense.

These are the exact words my tutor whispered after that first summer during which I began accompanying her to the cottage at Pine Lake.

I was terrified at first. It was one thing to sit at a semi-comfortable distance beside her at the kitchen table once a week, our books acting as our common denominator, but it was another thing altogether to consider spending an entire day and night with her, minus the security of school books between us. I estimated her age to be somewhere in the forties, and what could a forty-something-year-old woman and a twelve-year-old girl possibly find to do together in the span of twenty-four hours?

But my mother insisted.

You should feel honored, Honey. I don't expect she's got too many friends and she does seem to enjoy your company. So why not? School's out and the weather is grand. Besides it's only one night.

So I packed an extra pair of jeans, a sweatshirt, some warm pajamas and my rubber boots in case it should rain. My tutor came to collect me on a warm and lovely Friday afternoon in a two-tone green '57 Belair. I wondered why she had not driven to our tutoring sessions and said this aloud as we passed beneath the town's water tower and out towards the highway.

Your father said he'd drive me and I agreed. is all she had to say on the matter.

I didn't think you knew how to drive, I said.

To this she smiled, or grimaced. I was never sure which was which but took both to be a smile. I was more comfortable with smiles.

I am not quite as inept as most people like to think, is how she replied in a stilted tone.

We drove for a long while in silence. I watched the countryside whiz by through the side window, unsure how to conduct myself on this unprecedented journey. Did she expect me to proceed with the student-teacher mode, or was I to make an attempt at equalizing our relationship? Should I ask questions? Should I simply comment on the weather, as most adults seemed to do when nothing else came to mind? Or should I say nothing? I said nothing.

I had spent only one summer away from the prairies and every minute of that dragged-out summer I had longed to be back home on these dusty, southern prairies. Here you could see for miles in every direction, over patchwork fields; tuffs of shrubs; bursts of great branching elm or alder trees reaching out from the earth here and there, an anomaly amidst the flat, almost arid landscape. One could never feel congested or claustrophobic here as I had felt that one summer in the Rockies of British Columbia.

We whizzed past the grain elevator at Huxley, and up over the railway overpass. Below, less than a hundred yards from the track stood a dingy, colorless house badly in need of repair. From above, it looked like an abandoned playhouse, overgrown with weeds and discarded toys. The yard, encased in a high, chain-link fence was littered with a child's playthings, Tonka trucks, a tricycle, battered dolls, and so on. A scruffy, droopy-faced Saint Bernard, chained to the steps, raised its ears and sniffed the air as we passed by. This is when my tutor said something I didn't want her to say. What she said was too personal, bordering on indecent, for it permanently opened the window into her private life, a place I didn't even want to imagine at that point, a place of stifling solemnity that reeked of Lysol, lanolin and licorice; a place thick with the soundlessness of monotony and age; a graveyard of sorts, surrounded by dark, looming trees, overhanging a black iron fence with posts like spears pointing ominously upward into an infinitely gray sky.

She said this,

That house is like the one in which I grew up.

I was horrified! It was one thing to accept weekly canisters of Dutch licorice from this peculiar woman, but another thing to accept pieces of her private world. Whatever was I to do with it? I decided not to encourage her by simply not acknowledging this statement. We drove again for some time in silence. The landscape began to transform from flat, barren prairie into gatherings of trees - willows mainly, murky ponds, and smooth hilly terrain. At the Pine Lake turn-off, some twenty minutes hence, she spoke again as if there had been only a comma separating her last statement and the next.

Of course, it wasn't quite like that. Our house was made of bricks and mortar, one of the few like it in my village. But it was old and run down, like that old house back there under the tracks, and my younger brothers made such a mess in the yard that I was ashamed to admit I lived there, and it was set apart from the other houses, also near a railway track. We were very poor. During the war we dug up tulip bulbs from the garden, or anywhere we could find them, and my mother boiled them like potatoes. But after awhile there were no more tulip bulbs.

She didn't offer to tell me what was boiled in place of the tulip bulbs, which was fine because I was having a difficult time translating the information she'd already given me into a comprehensible image. For instance, I could not envision my tutor as a child, living amidst the ruins of a brick house with younger brothers to mess up the back yard. I was imagining those younger brothers as adults, male versions of my tutor, dressed in woolen trousers and tweed jackets, their hair glossed back with a ton of Brill Cream, tossing garbage about in the back yard, their mother bent over a hot stove in the kitchen furiously boiling tulips, bulbs, flowers and all, while bombs were exploding on everything but that brick house and its inhabitants. But I did have one imminent question:

Did you wear wooden shoes? is what I asked.

There was no mistaking the smile that stole over her tightly drawn face this time. She seemed pleased with my inquiry, thus, was I pleased with myself for asking.

Why yes, I did, as a matter of fact. Klompen, is what we call them. I still have a pair in my closet at home. I don't know why I have carted them about with me all these years. Perhaps, she paused, glancing down at my feet, *perhaps you would fit them. You will come to my house next week and try them on.* This was an order, it appeared, which I dared not defy.

There were a number of gates to be opened and closed. Although I did not volunteer for this task, when we pulled to a halt in front of the first of four, which was hidden amongst a row of pine trees, she said,

You'll find the latch on the other side. Just lift it off and swing the gate to the inside.

So this is what I did. We drove through what appeared to be a grazing pasture, judging by the great number of cow patties dotted about the hills, then came upon another gate. Instructions were given again, though in reverse order. This cycle repeated itself once more until we reached her two-acre lakefront property. One more gate and we were making our way slowly down a narrow lane, barely wide enough for her '57 Belair. Branches scraped at the sides, screeching like fingernails down a chalkboard. But she didn't flinch. She merely commented that things had become a tad disorderly since her last visit and perhaps she would find the hedge clippers and have me prune some of these trees. I was beginning to perceive that my fears of having nothing to do in the company of an exceedingly boring, older woman, were all but invalidated. I would be kept quite busy it seemed.

She'd never had company at the cottage before. She told me this as she was unlocking the door, me behind with an armload of kindling, which she had piled into my arms the moment I'd stepped out of the car.

She said it like this,

I've never wanted the bother of company out here. This place is my private domain. I have never allowed any intruders.

Her tone was somewhat threatening, as though this statement was a warning of sorts, an intimidation that let me know in no uncertain terms that I must tread lightly and mind my manners or I would be held responsible for stomping out her own personal nirvana forever.

I must have been expecting a stale-smelling, dark rodent hole for I was pleasantly surprised to find an uncluttered country cottage which smelled only faintly of Kerosene and Lysol. We entered directly into the kitchen area in which stood a chrome and white wood cooking stove, a drop-leaf table covered with a white lace tablecloth, two high-backed wooden chairs with woven seats and an open cupboard containing a sparse collection of mismatched kitchenware. There were two bedrooms, one on either side of the stove, separated by a wall, which didn't quite reach the ceiling. This was the cottage in its entirety, aside from a large screened verandah overlooking the lake. On the verandah stood a round wooden table and two more of the same sort of chairs. My tutor pointed to a cardboard kindling box just inside the verandah screen door into which I gratefully released my load.

Is that your boat? is what I asked her when I spotted the small blue and white rowboat bobbing at the end of a dock down at the water's edge.

Yes, it is, and we will go for a row later on, but you will come help unpack our things first, is what she ordered and I duly obeyed.

She had me take my suitcase into my designated room

and of course the first thing I did was to plop myself onto the springy mattress to see how much bounce I could muster out of it. But my childish frolic was short-lived for my tutor was only a step behind, carrying a set of flannel bed linen. After the beds were made, we made our way to the spring only a short distance away. I was delighted to find fresh sparkling water spurting out of the ground and dipped my face into it, gulping it down with gusto.

Come now, is what I heard her say with some impatience, above the gurgling of the water. *Work first, play later.*

We filled our pails and headed back.

My tutor brought out some sandwiches - ham and mustard, turkey and lettuce, and a pitcher of milk and set them on the white tablecloth.

You will find the dishes up there, she pointed towards the cupboard. *Please get two of everything. The cutlery is in the drawer underneath. And pull out the dish basin while you're there. I hope I have remembered to bring a new jar of dish soap. Later on we will take a walk by the lake.*

But we didn't. Neither of us had noticed the dark ring of clouds rising ominously from the eastern shore. While we dined we could hear the trees swaying lightly in a wind that seemed to have sprung up from nowhere. Before long the clouds began to spit rain, the wind gaining velocity and strength, the trees now visibly arching side to side, then a distant rumbling of thunder and seconds later, a flash across the sky, illuminating a thrashing lake and my tutor's little blue and white boat tossing mercilessly in the waves, banging up against the dock. Within minutes the storm was directly upon us. I rushed out onto the verandah excitedly. Each crash of thunder sounded as though the earth around us was bursting, shattering everything in its path.

Come now, urged my tutor in an overly calm voice. *We will get these dishes out of the way and have some tea. I believe the water is almost boiling. Please get the teapot from the cupboard, will you, and also a tea towel from the drawer,* which I did, though reluctantly.

Hot water was poured from the kettle into a basin of cold soapy water. The remainder of the hot water was poured into the teapot and set aside with two tea bags to steep. My tutor cleaned each plate thrice over while I waited, tea towel in hand. That's when I noticed that those big cumbersome hands of hers were visibly shaking. She knew, too, that I had taken note of this and these are the words she spoke in her calm, unwavering voice.

Thunder reminds me of the air raids. We have so many electrical storms here in Canada, especially here on the prairies. Often I wake suddenly at night ready to dive under my bed to take cover from the explosions. We were not actively involved in the war, you know. That is what is said, what is recorded. But it is not true. The war came to us whether we wanted it or not. We went hungry too. People died on our streets too - men, women, babies. Our men also went away and never came back.

Wars didn't matter much to me. Wars were things that happened in books with dates and names of important generals you had to remember for the exam. Wars happened in black and white. They sounded very dull, overrated. Still, I was curious about her part in it all. And so I asked,

When was the war?

Which one?

The one you were in.

A long time before you were born. I was only a child myself.

Where was the war?

The war was everywhere.

Was it here, too?

It was everywhere. We didn't all experience it in the same ways, but it was everywhere just the same.

We finished the dishes and sat down to our tea, both of us falling silent again as we gazed out onto the turbulent sky and lake. Before long the storm had moved on and the sun was once again beating down upon a glistening, revitalized earth.

Summer solstice had just passed and the nights were

warm and dusky until well after midnight. Around nine o'clock my tutor suggested we don our life jackets and take a short row around the inlet. She showed me how to brace my feet against the inside frame of the boat and with both arms, simultaneously lift the oars out of the water, thrusting my arms forward as the oars fell backwards, letting them slice through the lake's surface, then pulling my arms back towards my body. I was thrilled of course, exhilarated, when that little blue and white wooden boat began to ease gracefully through the water and I watched, spell-bound, as the shore line seemed to drift gracefully by.

We tried, each of us, taking an oar and rowing with concurrent efforts but her long, powerful arms were no match for my scrawny, still somewhat weakened, upper body. So we took turns at the helm, gliding past the shore, past other cottages, wharves, ski boats, canoes, and past the campground where campers had pitched tents and were roasting marshmallows over hot coals.

I was elated, watching the scenery drift lazily past. It was as though I had wings, no longer bound by the heaviness of my own limbs. I felt light and excitedly calm. There rose up something inside of me that wanted to shout and fall utterly silent both at once. I think my heart began to dance again that day after the last four months of aching weariness. And I owed it to my tutor, this great, stiff-haired lady in the bow of the boat whom I had once imagined a wicked and treacherous queen.

I chattered all the way home the next day, the wicked queen smiling shrewdly from behind the wheel, listening, seemingly pleased that she had broken through some unseen barrier.

The following Thursday she arrived at our door shortly after three o'clock. I was packed and waiting on the front step, barely able to contain my eagerness to set out in that blue and white row boat again. My tutor had agreed that I should bring my best friend, Wilma, and in fact, I thought I detected a covert twinkle of delight behind those sparkly glasses although her actions and tone of voice revealed complete imperviousness.

Wilma also, was waiting restlessly on the front verandah, and came bounding across the lawn, pigtails bouncing off her shoulders the minute we'd pulled into the yard. Wilma's mother stood in the front doorway, wiping her hands on her apron and waving,

Yous girls have a good time now and don't go pestering anybodys too much.

My tutor appeared to be satisfied with her decision to allow Wilma and I to accompany her another half dozen times to the lake that summer. It required less effort on her part to keep us entertained. The lake, the little blue and white boat and the many trails through the bush were, to two twelve-year-old girls, an endless playground. She did not allow us to be idle either, and by the end of the summer her trees were well pruned back from the narrow lane, the cottage and dock were repainted, and annual flowers bloomed from every inch of earth surrounding the cottage.

It was mid August. I had awakened in that metal bed with an uncomfortably full bladder. Early morning light was peering in fluted columns through the lacy curtains, but it was too early to rise for a full day. Blearily, I crawled over Wilma, who was still sleeping soundly, her freckled face serene with oblivion, pulled on my rubber boots and tramped to the outhouse. On my way back in through the screened verandah something caught my attention. Something moving down at the end of the dock. I stopped and turned to look, rubbing my blurry eyes.

What I witnessed that early August morning made me gasp inwardly and I hurriedly entered the verandah, easing the door shut behind me so that it wouldn't creak. I wakened Wilma and we tiptoed out to the verandah. There on the dock was the figure of a completely nude woman, her back towards us. She was sitting on the edge of the dock, dangling her feet in the water. Then she turned and lowered herself gracefully into the water, her mouth open in quick gasps as her body penetrated the cool water. Wilma and I poked one another, suppressing our giggles. But the thrill wore off in a matter of seconds. I don't know exactly how Wilma was feeling at that moment, but as I watched my naked tutor down there, basking in the chilly early morning sun, it was as though that long, lithe body of hers was emitting a subtle glow, an aura of near perfection, and all at once I felt like I was looking into the face of God and had to turn away in my own unworthiness.

We crawled back into bed, pulled the covers up over our heads and were soon asleep again. When we awoke, the sun was pouring in through the curtained window and my tutor was bustling about in the kitchen, stoking the stove, pouring hot water into the teapot. She was, of course, fully clothed in her pleated wool skirt, beige leotards and white cashmere sweater. It was as if that early morning revelation had been but a dream and so I thought little more about it.

It was Wilma who, unwittingly, let me in on the gossip that began flitting around our uptight little prairie town. She'd heard it from her elder brother who'd heard it from his circle of friends and, before too long, it was circulating throughout the entire town. It was improper, they were saying, that a middle-aged woman should be taking two little girls out into the woods, alone, with her. There were stronger, more descriptive adjectives like, *filthy, perverted, obscene, pornographic, pedophile* - words for which I had no definitions back then.

In my eager innocence I petitioned my tutor to take Wilma and I on one last trip to the cottage before the fall school term began. She bent her head low, for we had met up in the drug store in the shampoo section, and this is what she said in a hoarse whisper,

I don't think so, though I don't know why I should say so. Why should I defend myself? I have no need of defense.

I hadn't known then what she meant.

Now I know only too well.

shshshshshshshshshshsh

As I rumble into the garage on the quad I am thinking that I have way too much time to think. I spend too much time alone, but people wear me out and I end up desperately wanting solitude, so what am I to do? I am caught, but not in a web. I am caught in a void of nothingness. I am not allowed the security of a web, the security of knowing my fate. Sometimes I am not on the inside looking out, but on the outside looking in. I am out here where there is no form, no viable order, nothing in which to contain oneself. All the parts of me are roaming about out here, colliding now and then, bumping off each other like bumper cars. There is no gravity, no magnetic field to force myself into tidy bubbles like everything else in this universe. But what am I to do?

I must get myself together if I am to take that walk down to the river today. I am almost bursting with anticipation. My senses get ahead of me somehow. I have already imagined how the river will look, smell, taste and sound today. I must feel it.

Peeling away some of the layers of clothing after stepping into the house, I set my boots neatly on the mat, fold my clothes and put them away in the closet. I am ignoring the drowsiness. Mind over matter, remember?

I pull a moose roast out of the freezer, place it in the microwave on high while I scrub six potatoes, peel four carrots and an onion, which makes me cry. I open the microwave and remove the hunk of meat which is partially cooked now on one

69

side, and chuck it into the slow cooker with a package of Lipton's onion soup mix as any good housewife ought to do. I cut up the potatoes, slice the carrots and onions, pour in a cup of water, replace the lid, plug it in, switch it on to high.

A dull ache in my spine causes me to tense up. The pain worsens with every move, every breath. Mind over matter. Matter over mind. Before I take that walk I should lie down for a bit, maybe half an hour, concentrate on relaxing my muscles. But I can't leave the kitchen in disarray. Carrot and onion peelings get swiped up and tossed into a bucket for the chickens later. The counter gets wiped down. I lean over the counter while I work, stretching out my back, breathing steadily. Pain in my knees and ankles is rendering them weak. They tremble.

First, the dishes must be done. The plug gets put in place, soap dribbled in, hot water tap turned on. The dirty dishes get gathered up and placed into the sink. A clean cloth is retrieved from the linen drawer. My head wants to fall off my shoulders onto the floor and the rest of me wants to go with it. My body becomes heavier with every breath, until the last dish is set into the drainer. No, first I must wipe out the sink. I mustn't relax until everything is in its place.

At last I stumble into the bedroom, pull back the blankets and crawl inside. Once I have lain down, the muscles of this wretched body begin to relax, and that's when I become fully aware of the pain. It is ripping through my chest. I struggle with every breath. It feels like there is a two hundred pound weight crushing my legs, my arms. Then my legs begin to jump and twitch. My doctor says it is exhaustion, which causes this, another syndrome.

Restless leg syndrome is what she calls it. *Chronic Fatigue Syndrome. Leaky Gut Syndrome, Fibromyalgia Syndrome. Irritable Bowel Syndrome. Irritable Bladder Syndrome. Irritable Esophagus Syndrome.* Irritable Everything Syndrome.

If it would do any good, I would cry. But it doesn't, so I won't. If it would do any good to pray, I would. But it doesn't, not that I've ever noticed anyway. Where is God? Where is that great, loving, caring, faceless head in the sky who looks down on us with tenderness and tends to all our needs, who cares for the sparrow? Where are those giant hands with the holes in them that beckon,

Come unto me all ye who are weary and heavy laden and I will give thee rest?

Oh God! God! *God*! *GOD*! Could it be true what they say? Could it be that I am being punished? Or that God refuses to hear me cry because I am iniquitous? What have I done, and could I undo it?

When I was young, that spring I fell ill, I used to pray. I made deals with God and would have done anything if only He would take away my tummy ache, the heavy throbbing in my legs, or my headache. I would sweep and scrub the kitchen linoleum nearly down to the sub-floor. I would take a pale of soapy water and wash the bathroom, floor to ceiling, even the toilet, with my bare hands. I washed windows, polished the piano, brushed and scraped the dandruff from my mother's hair. I would tell my father I loved him, which I truly did. I would bring him his slippers and slide them onto his knobby feet. I would bake him chocolate cakes, which he loved because they were a scrumptious change from my mother's carob brownies. I did everything my mother told me to, almost. I pleaded with God. It appeared that I was keeping my end of the bargain and that God was not. But after-all, it was my bargain. Not His.

Yes, eventually I entered a period of remission for a time, but not because I'd prayed. Funny thing is, I haven't given up. It is as though I still believe I will be healed. My husband prays too. His prayers are simple, earnest, and to the point. He cries sometimes. He gets right down on his knees, lays his head in my lap, wraps his long, heavy arms around my waist and cries with such sincerity that I want to cry too,

God, please make my wife well!

My first husband prayed also. But his prayers were much different. He prayed for my obedience. He prayed that if need be God would chastise me to bring me back to the fold. He prayed that I would become the ideal pastor's wife. Instead, I divorced him. Whatever was I thinking, becoming a pastor's wife? I couldn't even play the piano!

It went something like this:

During our seventeenth summer, Wilma and I headed for the coast where would we spend the summer at a camp out on Quadra Island. Wilma would be a counselor, but I, deprived of siblings, did not think I would suit a cabin full of grimy, demanding children. Instead I chose the kitchen. I was well versed in kitchen duty.

We clambered aboard the train in Edmonton, rode wide-eyed through the night, through the mountains and the interior of British Columbia. From Vancouver we took the ferry across to Victoria where we caught the greyhound up-island to Campbell River. A crew from the camp met us there. We stayed a night on a church floor. I slept under a grand piano, Wilma, on a pew. In the morning we set out by boat, with our luggage, to the island.

Only a week into the summer, that old familiar body ache seemed to be returning. It was barely perceptible, but it was there. That dull ache in my spine, the heaviness in my limbs, queasiness in my gut. I did not fight it, but neither did I acknowledge it. Instead I simply retired to my room earlier in the evenings than the others and spent my free time alone, rather than in games with some of the other staff. I tried to ignore it.

We met on the second day. He was hitching a boat to the dock and I was on a break. He said this,

You have the most mysterious eyes. Let me look at them.

And this is what he did. He looked into my eyes. But I am at fault because I allowed him to do this. He grasped my tingling hand and took me a way through the trees, along the island's rocky shore until we came upon an old boat that had run aground many years before and no one had bothered with it since. It was too old for repair, the wood beginning to rot through. The boat's name was Goforth. This beautifully fitting name was etched into the exterior surface of the cabin above the hatchway. The cabin's interior was, for the most part, still intact, although some of the wallboards had cracked in many places. There was a single bunk attached to a small wooden table and some enclosed shelving along one wall. When I stepped from the dock onto this magnificent craft I instantly thought of my tutor's blue and white rowboat. I wanted to take the Goforth out into the water and feel that winged lightness again, the air streaming through my hair, the shore moving dreamily past. I wanted to come unstuck from the earth.

I have never seen such a pretty lady, is what my new friend commented inside the Goforth's cabin.

Neither have I, is what I said, not realizing at first he'd meant me, not the boat. I was touching the walls, running my fingers down the textured surface where the varnish had peeled down to a thin, flaky, yellowed layer. The boat swayed slightly in the water. I closed my eyes, something I shouldn't have done.

He said, touching my lips with his fingertips,

I have never seen such beautiful lips.

I guessed then that he wasn't referring to the Goforth and opened my eyes, moving swiftly towards the exit. It wasn't that I wanted to get away from him or his touch, for I didn't. It was the unfamiliarity that I wanted to escape. He apologized.

Forgive me. It's just that you are so very intriguing and I wasn't expecting to be intrigued by anything while I was up here this summer. Not much will catch my eye the way that you have. I hope you'll allow me to get to know you?

This seemed all right with me. I relayed the incident to Wilma that evening in my room, the two of us perched cross-legged on my bed.

Oh! she exclaimed, clutching her hands to her heart, her

chin raised, eyes fluttering theatrically. *How did you do it? Don't you know that he's the apple in every girl's eye? I could name ten girls right now who would give their left arm to have him say those things to them!*

It was then that I began to realize how critical physical appearances were. He had raven hair, cropped short above his ears; a wide, circular, but symmetrical, face; an obvious shadow over his upper lip, chin and cheeks which suggested a certain desirable maturity. He was stocky, but toned, barrel-chested, and had a smooth, level voice, which did seem to make some of the girls run off giggling when he spoke. He dressed himself in crisp, new blue jeans and red suspenders over white t-shirts, and wore brown clogs on his feet, which, on any other man, might have appeared effeminate, but on him, they were simply icing on the cake.

Halfway through the summer, after we had spent much time together, he said this to me,

In three years I want to marry you. Could you promise me that you'll come back in three years and marry me?

It seemed like an acceptable solution to the problem of what to do with my life. Most of the other girls had already charted their education paths, careers, marriages with or without children, even retirement. This fairly handsome man was asking me to wait for him while he completed his Bible School training and got himself set up somewhere behind a church pulpit. I could be a preacher's wife. I liked going to church. I liked the holy feeling I would get after everyone else had gone and I remained hidden between two of the pews. Somebody would turn the lights off and it would become so quiet and still I would feel like the whole world had stopped except me, and if I should give the directive, the world would begin again, but only at my command. I prayed a lot in church too. I thought that God might be more receptive to my supplication if it came from a church pew. Perhaps this was my atonement. If I were to marry this preacher man and carry on the duties of a devout preacher's wife, then God would have no choice but to listen to me.

And so I said, *Okay.*

My mother was hysterical, happy, anxious, aghast, relieved, worried, and so on. My father told me I was too young.

But I suppose, in three years you won't be quite so young, will you? is what he said, cuddling me in his furry arms.

I'd been given a promise ring by that aspiring preacher man, but very soon, I wearied of thrusting my left hand before of all the other girls' astonished faces. We still had two more years of high school left.

Wilma grew ardently studious during those final years of school. Yet she seemed to breeze through each class with the effortlessness of a soaring eagle. But by the time school was out for the day, all I wanted was a hot bath and my bed. I believe that I lost my sense of objectivity during those years. Did I become a social recluse because my aching, fatigued body dictated my social life? Or did I fall ill because the pressures and demands that other people placed upon me were more stimulation than my temperate disposition could handle?

So she whizzed past me, Wilma and my other classmates. I watched them go, one by one, some of them slowly but with dogged determination, others with the speed and agility of a Tasmanian devil. But what could I do? While they gabbed in their exclusive, enthusiastic circles about boys, about university, about hair and make-up and fashions, I was alone in my bedroom writing letters back and forth to my fiancé.

We both graduated at the same time, he from seminary, and I, from high school. I did not leave the podium with an advanced diploma, not even honors. I emerged from those twelve years with a scroll of paper tied with a blue ribbon. My classmates partied for the entire weekend. Most of them wouldn't remember anything after being handed their declaration of accomplishment. I went home and packed. My mother cried and blew her nose. My father sat in his easy chair, elbows on knees, with his whiskered chin in the palms of his hands and sighed.

My fiancé had decided that things would go better for him with a wife by his side. Churches wanted a married man, untempted by the young girls in the church, an experienced man who could speak to them of marriage. So we married a year before we'd initially planned and settled in Nanaimo on a three-acre plot, my husband still searching for church pastorship.

Within only a month of marriage, he decided things might go better for him if his wife was pregnant. Churches wanted a family man, stable with family responsibilities, one who could speak to them of family matters. A man principled and virile, fruitful and actively multiplying the earth with his quiver-full of children. Within a few short months, my belly was beginning to sprout. I was nineteen years old.

We were accepted into a small community church less than a mile from our home. This way, the neighbors could catch a satisfactory glimpse of the local pastor and his virtuous wife taking obligatory strolls on a Saturday evening, and early to the church on Sunday mornings. There were also Tuesday evening prayer meetings, Wednesday missionary meetings, Thursday youth group meetings and Friday family nights.

My preacher husband made love to me on Monday nights, for it was the only night during the week, which was not cluttered with a flurry of church activities. He was considerate in that he always asked permission first. I never declined, for I accepted this, with neither complaint nor desire, as one of my wifely duties. He was not rough or brusque in his lovemaking, but neither was he gentle or eager to satisfy me. I think he believed that my satisfaction was in the giving of pleasure. This was true, to an extent, although there were times when I secretly longed for the gentle caresses he had lavished upon me during our two-year, long distance courtship by telephone or mail. Plus, I did not give so much as he just helped himself.

We made love only at night with the curtains drawn and the bedroom door locked as though he thought someone might just waltz right into our house, unannounced, and come right into our bedroom. This was not an entirely unrealistic fear as church patrons often did show up on our doorstep, but so far, no one had ventured into the privacy of our bedroom.

Sometimes he would watch me undress, undistracted by Bibles or concordances or pads of paper and pen for sudden inspirations, and I would feel as though he were scanning his stores of cognitive rationale for a justification of his lust for me. Sometimes he would undress me, unbuttoning my blouse and sliding it from my shoulders with an histrionic flare as though we were both actors and spectators in the drama. He would unhook my bra and remove it with deliberate precision, never fumbling. Our clothing never got tossed about carelessly, but was scrupulously laid out on the bedside table or the vanity bench. He would ask whether I wanted to be on top or on the bottom as though he were doing me a great favor by asking. And though it never really mattered to me where I was, I would concede to making this decision, as it appeared to be my only contribution to our conjugal life.

Most of the time he would cover my body completely with his. He would wrap both of his legs around me so that my lower half was completely immobile, and grasp my hands in his, raising them onto the pillows so that we formed the crude silhouette of an angel. He would start out slowly, methodically, but within minutes, would gain momentum until it seemed he had forgotten who or what was beneath him, like I was little more than a hole in the mattress. His rhythmic huffing and moaning also made it seem as though this was an onerous chore, more grueling work than shoveling snow in a prairie winter, and nowhere near as revitalizing and invigorating. Near the finale his voice would begin to rise in tone and intensity until at last, he would let out a high-pitched squeal.

God! GOD! he would shout in much the same way I say it when my pain has gone beyond belief. His entire body would shudder and he would lie there, on top of me, a quivering, panting mass of spent flesh.

I took pride in my ability to bring him to these pathetic depths of uncontrollable expulsions. The greatest satisfaction I stole from our lovemaking was in this secret, undeclared ascendancy I held over him. In fact, I wanted him much more than one night a week. To hold him, utterly helpless, in my female clutches, was the only means of control in my world of constant duty and demand. But not once did I use or manipulate this mastery. I held it inside where it kept me smug and warm during those times when I was just a wife, just a polite smile or handshake. During his sermons when every eye and ear was intent upon my God-fearing, preacher husband's antics up there behind the pulpit, I took a sort of perverse comfort in knowing that I could disarm that well-groomed persona of perfect control and make him yelp in such an unmasculine, undignified manner. I could make him take the Lord's name in vain. I could make him forget God.

Our son was born in May. He was born screaming at me and he never stopped.

I didn't make a very good pastor's wife after-all. Not only could I not play the piano, I often fell asleep during my husband's sermons and he would have to rouse me quickly during the benediction so that I could grasp his arm and accompany him to the foyer where we would show our teeth and grip hands with all the members of our little flock. During the Tuesday night prayer meetings, I would become so restless that I would get up out of my pew and pace about in the back. Sometimes I snuck a book into the Wednesday night missionary meetings, placing it between the pages of my open Bible, devouring the fascinating, often disturbing, stories of Ray Bradbury or Edgar Allen Poe. After our son was born I was excused from the Thursday night youth meetings, but Friday family nights I was to be a shining epitome of family unity. I wasn't, of course. My son raced around punching all of the other children, making them holler and rush for their mothers' skirts, and I did nothing to stop him. My legs were faint with pain and stiffness. I was always congested and had a constant sore throat so that I really did not want to talk to anyone except for the donkey I had bought for twenty-five dollars whose name was Will because he had the coloring and temperament of my best friend, Wilma.

Finally, one evening, my preacher husband carted our son off to his bedroom and left him screeching in his crib, after telling me he needed to have a word with me. A chair was pulled up in front of me where I had been reading on the sofa, the book was taken sternly from my hands, and then he looked into my eyes not at all in the same way he had first looked at them on board the Goforth, when he had commented on how very mysterious and beautiful they were.

Why are you staring at me? is what I asked, wearily gearing up for a battle I wasn't prepared to fight.

I am looking into your soul, he said in a disturbingly gentle manner. *You know very well that you are making a mockery of my ministry. I am a leader. Leaders lead. What I need is a helpmate, a wife who supports my leadership, not one who hinders it. What do you do for the church? Do you attend the ladies' group? Do you teach Sunday school? Do you do anything at all besides sit here and read or talk to that blasted ass out there? Your son is a disgrace, your actions appalling.*

I tried to apologize. I tried to agree. But I couldn't. Tears began to squirt from my eyes and I sobbed this instead,

I'm tired. I don't feel well. My legs hurt. My head pounds. My gut always aches. I'm constipated. I have diarrhea. My fingers don't work. I have cramps. I'm bleeding fourteen days out of the month. My breasts hurt. My face hurts. I haven't enough breath in me to talk. I really, really don't feel well!

Well, if you ask me, I'd say that if you would just quit telling yourself that you're sick, you wouldn't be. It's as simple as that, no ifs, buts, or ands. You've been to the doctor. There is nothing wrong with you. It's all in your head and you're going to have to deal with that. I am not asking you to shape up. I am telling you.

I believed him. I believed that I was just lazy, so I tried harder. I really did. I went to the ladies' group. I baked for raffles and charities. I tended the church nursery twice a month. I entertained guests in my home, made a bazillion pots of coffee, a thousand pot roasts. Missionaries that came through on their furloughs emptied their suitcases in our spare bedroom. Their children stunk up my bathroom, tracked mud through my halls. I endured my husband's surliness every Saturday night when his sermons weren't quite coming together the way he wished, and watched him transform into the amiable, proficient preacher that his congregation knew by ten a.m. the next morning.

My husband's prayers at home went like this,

Great Father in Heaven, make this family strong. Give my wife a spirit of giving and selflessness. Free her from this bondage of sin that hinders her testimony for You, and so on.

But instead of freedom from my bondage of sin, I became depressed, hopelessly immersed in my own secluded world of bone-wearying exhaustion. During Friday family night, I would slouch off into a corner alone and would put such a miserable look on my face that no one dared tread anywhere within five yards of me. Pain in my back and legs prevented me from sleeping during the Sunday morning services, but sitting up for more than ten minutes had become an unbearable feat so I would tuck my head into the cradle of my arms on the pew in front of me and pose there until my preacher husband descended from the podium, grasping my aching arm and dragging me with him to the vestibule where I would put on a dazed, but dutiful, smile. At home I quit eating those juicy pot roasts for I'd learned that if I had to sit up and entertain, it was easier and less uncomfortably carried out on an empty stomach.

Eventually my preacher husband suggested that I seek the advice of a psychiatrist. He said I needed to be medicated. He didn't say it quite like that. This is what he said,

You are going to see a shrink. People like you either need to be hospitalized or on medication. I can't believe it has come to this. But I will personally see to it that you get help. Neither I nor my congregation deserves to suffer because of your mental problems. We have let this go on far too long and its time to stop now.   He did not say this unkindly, but more matter-of-factly, as one might be told to don a raincoat because it was raining.

The doctor asked me a whole lot of questions which I can't remember now, and had me go through a half dozen quizzes, puzzles, picture defining, story-telling and so on. This whole shamozzle took about six hours.   I was so utterly exhausted afterwards that I curled up into a ball, as tight as I could squeeze myself and refused to budge from that hospital evaluation room. So they found a bed for me in a semi-private room on the psychiatric ward, sedated me with some sort of brown bitter-tasting liquid in a Styrofoam cup and I slept for two days, or maybe more.

It is difficult now, looking back through time, which is blurred by murky waves and emotional debris, to impose any kind of judgment on this particular interval of my life. I did so want to please my preacher husband, and all he wanted was a normal wife, so this is what my head aspired to be. But my body had other agendas and the two separate entities fought like territorial coons.   When I awoke from that dreamless, colorless, medicated sleep, I saw that my forearms were bandaged up in white gauze and I became so frightened that I began flailing about but quickly realized also that my arms were stuck. Someone had secured them to the metal railing of my bed. I was completely constrained to a hospital bed.

It took almost a week for that doctor to come back with all of my test results.

You are clearly in a state of deep depression, is what he told me, reading from the chart in his lap, then raising his dark, unsmiling eyes to me. *We will start you on a medication, but you should know that it sometimes takes up to six weeks for it to begin to work, and in the meantime, you may feel a little dizzy, edgy, perhaps even a little more depressed. But we'll monitor this closely. You won't be alone, I promise you that.*

He patted my arm, still bruised and crusty from where

I'd try to slash myself, mindlessly, in my sleep. A kind of flat tenderness could be detected in his voice and in his brief, heartfelt touch. This simple gesture gave me just one more reason to get better. I determined right then that I would do everything this doctor told me, no mistakes. I would get well.

I also believe you have anorexia and we will address this immediately. You will be assigned a nurse who will draw up a care plan for you. She, or he, will stay with you during mealtimes and for one hour afterward to make sure you don't purge. But remember, it's up to you. You have to fight.

There was no more fight in me. All I wanted to do, at that point, was sleep. But fight I would, if that's what was required.

And one more thing, he said, slipping his pen back into his breast pocket. *We evaluated your IQ level, though you probably weren't aware of this. You scored in the top three percent.*

Three dizzying weeks later, my preacher husband, who had visited me dutifully every day as though I was merely one of his flock, came to retrieve me from the hospital. He wasn't unpleasant, but neither was he overly agreeable. He simply said,

Well I hope things will go better now.

I took the drugs, every day, like clockwork, enduring the dizziness, the jitteriness, burred vision, nausea and drowsiness, in the hopes of attaining appropriate heights of pastor's wifeship. The congregation was sympathetic and allowed me the privilege of opting out of the weekly meetings. All that was required of me was wakefulness on Sunday mornings and a few pot roasts during the week. This meant I had more time to spend outside in the small corral I had built for Will, who nuzzled his fuzzy nose in my neck and did absolutely nothing else I wanted him to.

After another year of this my preacher husband handed me a bus ticket and told me to leave our son with his sister and go home to visit my parents.

A rest might smarten you up, is what he sighed.

For the first week of my visit back home on the prairies, I slept. My mother had kept my attic bedroom in a mausoleum-like preservation. She fussed over me and bulk shopped at the health food store again. My father smiled a lot and patted my shoulders, unsure if it was acceptable to hug another man's wife. Wilma was still in Calgary in her third year of nursing and only a handful of my other classmates remained.

My first outing back home was to my tutor's house. Her horn-rimmed glasses had been replaced with a pair of wide plastic ones. This was the only change I could detect upon first glance. She greeted me at the door in her pleated woolen skirt, beige leotards and white cashmere sweater. Her hair was just as stiff and dull as ever and her large, uncomely hands reached out in greeting as I entered. She had never before made such an intimate gesture, but after two years of routine hand-shaking in the church vestibule, it did not occur to me that she was extending herself to me in a way she had never offered herself to anyone.

It was not a chastisement, what she said to me while sipping our tea that day. Her words were merely reflections of her own experience, which I softly integrated into my own. She said this,

People can force us into words or behaviors that we would not, under other circumstances, say or do. But no matter what, we are always in charge of how we feel. No one can dictate the attitude we choose to take in any particular situation.

Do you think I have been wrong then, to feel the way I do?

It is not up to me to voice an opinion. I don't know how you feel. All I do know is that you are capable of choosing. During the war our village was ravaged, not just by the Germans, but by our own efforts of resistance. I remember the

day the government called for the mobilization of our units. Because we lived so near the railroad, our home became a sort of central station. Eventually we were forced out of our own home so that it could be used as a station. Mamma and Pappa took us four children to a boarding house that was already crowded with refugees, many of them Jews, heading for the coast in the hopes of escape. I remember the stench of all those people under one roof. We tried to keep the children indoors when the bombing began but it was virtually impossible to keep track of them all.

Holland was taking out its own dikes, flooding the land in an attempt to delay the German army. But they did not come by land. They came by air. We were huddling in a makeshift room behind an upstairs bedroom wall when we heard the news crackling over our illegal radio. Rotterdam had been taken out, an entire city in one blast. I remember shrinking away from the rest of the group, feeling ill and hopeless. I wanted my life to end. I did not want to live in a world where men killed each other without thought or conscience.

Holland surrendered then, but it only worsened our lot. Every able male was taken by force into German manpower. They would roar into town and take, at gunpoint if need be, every man in view and would search the houses for whom they considered the cowards. Pappa was among those taken from our house. He, and about a dozen others, some only boys of fourteen, maybe younger. But Mamma wouldn't let him go without a fuss, as always. She ran after him, clawing and biting the German soldiers. I saw this with my own eyes from the shed where we and some other women were taking cover with the children. She jumped on the back of one of the soldiers and bit his neck. It might have been funny under other circumstances, although what other circumstance could there be that would have provoked her to the point of such violence? She was screaming and Pappa was wide-eyed, calling at her to hush and go back to tend to the children. Everything would turn out okay, he called back. Everything would be okay.

Such a commotion she was causing in her fury that the

soldier turned and kicked her in the belly. But she did not relent. It was only fuel to her fire. I saw him take his rifle, cock it and point it at her head. I saw his finger on the trigger. It was almost as if I was seeing in slow motion what took place in only a matter of seconds. Then I saw Mamma's head blow right off her shoulders and bounce onto the ground inside the fence, and I saw the rest of her body stumble a moment, then collapse. One of my younger brothers went running out to her. He was shot down, too, in the confusion, only a foot away from Mamma. One of the soldiers shouted something in German and another one grabbed ahold of her legs and dragged her to a nearby ditch. But my little brother and Mamma's head still lay there in pools of blood. I saw Pappa's eyes as they thrust him into the truck and sped away. We never saw him again. His eyes, though, I remember his eyes.

She quietly sipped on her tea for a few moments, then went on.

I remember feeling that I just couldn't go on. I couldn't imagine a peaceful world after that. So many people in our village were sick. Many of them died from hunger. But I had my two younger brothers to look after. If I were to die, who would look after them? I even considered taking them with me. I considered fastening ropes around their little necks and mine. But I couldn't do it. They were so innocent. They didn't know there was a war going on. They didn't even know what had happened to Mamma. I was only eight years old. But I decided, then, that I would be strong. I pushed aside thoughts of our wicked world and did not give in to the torment. Yes, I was in pain, such pain as cannot be described, as was everyone. But pain became my motivation. As long as I had pain I could survive. I decided, then, to raise my two brothers and live to be an old lady.

shshshshshshshshshsh

I drove myself back to the island only to collect my few possessions and my son. But when I saw my two-year-old playing quietly by himself, not destroying everything in his path as I was used to seeing him, I backed out of the bedroom and shut the door, pausing. My sister-in-law shrugged her shoulders and said,

He's been like this ever since you left except when his daddy comes once a week. Other than that, he's no trouble whatsoever. I can't explain it, but he seems happy. Why don't you just leave him for awhile? It's no trouble, really.

My preacher husband had little to say regarding my decision, except to reiterate that I was the downfall of his ministry.

You would choose to destroy my life's work like this? he said, his stocky figure darkening the doorway while I packed. *Everything I have worked towards, my entire life?*

No, I would not choose to do anything of the sort. But what I do choose, is to be in control of my own life and my own feelings. What you do with yours is your business, not mine.

But I thought we were a team. We were in this together. Don't you remember? You said you wanted to be in the ministry with me. Remember that? We're a team, husband and wife. We're a family. Doesn't that count? What God has joined together let no man put asunder.

You are not a husband. You are a master and you wish

86

me to be your servant, and I don't think that's what that means. Besides, I don't even like you.

That was all I had to say so I left him standing there, a puzzled look of confusion and despair pervading his round face. As I walked away from him I could sense the heat mounting behind me, his face contorting, reddening with anger, desperation, disbelief. He would be running his broad hands through his black hair. He would be staring through the air, in my direction, but not at me. His eyes would be unfocused, just like all those Saturday nights when he would pace the floor in his study, searching for the appropriate idiom, the correct emotion, to be paired with the correct word, the right clench or wave of fist, or the suitable facial expression or bodily gesture. But this time, all those years of theology would prove to be worthless, as they had only prepared him to deal with other people's troubles, not his own.

I did not mean to be petulant or rude and I most certainly did not wish him any harm. The knowledge that my preacher husband would be wallowing in self-pity and misery because of me was almost more than I could bear. I considered turning back, at least to try to explain. I would have liked to spell it all out for him in a language he could understand. But we did not speak the same language. I would have liked to touch his face, my fingers lightly pressing against his brow, his cheeks. I would have liked for him to accept this modest caress in exchange for my freedom. But to turn back now would only prolong the agony for both of us.

It wasn't his fault. I loved him. I truly did and I wanted more than anything to be his partner, an equal partner, to grow with him into old age. He wasn't exactly unkind. He just didn't quite get it. But how could I expect him to understand when no one else could? I didn't even understand myself. I believed I was lazy and depressed and unhappy, just like he, and many others, told me. I went away from him because I thought it would be better for everyone if I was lazy, depressed and unhappy on my own time, on my own turf.

Heading northward along the coast, my windshield wipers steadily beating time against the pattering of rain on the windshield, spraying out behind the tires, I began to become aware of the utter futility of my life. My preacher husband and my only son were back there somewhere living their lives without me. Or I was living my life without them. Why couldn't I have kept pace? Others managed it, and managed well. If human beings could live through the unthinkable, deprecating torment of concentration camps then why could I not brace myself against the every day meager demands of family or clergy life? If people could shovel excrement, splashing it onto themselves without wincing; if they could manage to slumber nine men to a six-and-a-half-by-eight bed made of raw boards, immobile, two blankets per bed; if they could walk miles through ice and snow in bare feet; if they could watch and breathe the stench of smoke floating in heavy columns from the chimneys of crematoriums - then why, oh why could I not cheerfully endure a little bit of weariness? Was this even a comparable allusion?

In Campbell River I hired a youth of about seventeen to ferry me over to Quadra. I thanked him, paid him what I could and asked him to return for me the next day at the same time. My mission, of course, was to set the Goforth afloat again, me with it. It was a foolish notion. More than foolish, quite completely absurd. Even if the motor had been in running condition, I would not have known how to operate it. There were two rather eroded paddles on board, but I could not have maneuvered that boat by myself with only two paddles. And last, even if I untied it from the wharf and somehow freed it from the rocky floor of the bay and set it afloat, I would have no way of getting back to shore – if I'd wanted to, that is.

Nonetheless, rather than sit there on the old pier scolding myself for drastically overrating my capabilities, I stepped out onto the Goforth expecting to be immediately transformed into that light-winged, celestial being that had possessed me all those years ago when my tutor had first set my eager hands upon the oars of her blue and white row boat.

It didn't happen, of course. There was no transformation, only the irregular lapping of salt water against the warped, wooden sides of the Goforth, the steady cries of gulls and the distant splashing of sea lions surfacing, plunging and re-surfacing again and again.

From the bow I gazed out over the bay, over the numerous islands, both rocky and lush, dotting the seascape, and far off into the horizon where gray waters blended into gray sky, neither distinguishable from the other. I wished for wings to soar with the gulls. I wished for the sleek agility of the sea lions to glide, without restraint, through both sky and sea. I even wished for the certainty, the plenitude, of the forests, through placid or stormy weather. I wished to be that singular rock on the bluff high above me, overhanging land and sea as though it were the fearsome, immortal god of both. I watched as the wavering horizon swallowed up the last bright swirl of sun, leaving behind muted streaks of melon, rose and indigo.

All that night I laid there, shivering, on a bare, cold bunk inside the Goforth's cabin, imagining what it must have been like to have fished from the edges of this boat, out there amidst the rolling blue-gray waves of the bay. I imagined what it might have been like to have been a fish, caught and struggling in a net, tugged up over the sides of this boat, flailing on the deck, gills flapping in desperation, gasping and choking, dying. I imagined that I was a pirate with only one eye, a sword in its sheath at my side, ready to slash anything or anyone who attempted to oppose me. I imagined that I had guts, strong and sturdy enough to hold out through the worst tempest.

I imagined myself asleep, rocking peacefully in my tutor's little blue and white rowboat.

shshshshshshshshshsh

I know now that I won't be taking any mile walk down to
the river today. Maybe tomorrow. Tomorrow I will be more
careful. I will spend more time in my waking exercises and
will drink the liquid from two juice boxes through a straw
before I rise from my bed, as my wise and learned doctor tells
me I should. I will get up more slowly. I will walk more
slowly, breathe more deeply. I will concentrate on conserving
every bit of precious energy so that I will be well enough to
walk that distance.

The aroma of simmering stew stirs my hunger pangs,
which gnaw at my gut. Oh, I am so famished sometimes, but
am too afraid to eat more than a couple of bites at a time. Even
a spoonful of cereal will clog up my insides and I will feel
intense lethargy, severe bloating and pain around my middle. I
have learned that the satisfaction of swallowed food is not
worth the physical distress or the emotional frustration it
almost, invariably, causes. I eat only in very modest quantities,
carefully and consciously chewing each bite so that it will mix
with digestive juices from my saliva glands all the way down
through my intestines, instead of leaking out through the
intestinal walls, provoking an attack by my own immune
system.

It is now almost two o'clock in the afternoon. I have
wasted yet another day. What did I do wrong? And why do I
continue to blame myself? Have I not yet accepted that there
is not a single thing I can do about it? Always, I look for some

90

excuse, some pattern, a misjudgment perhaps - something I can avoid or modify in the future. I have avoided refined sugar, thinking that this was the culprit. It is torturous, denying myself those rapturous sweets, which taste so divine on the tongue but become muddy slugs in my intestines. I have avoided wheat and other grains, thinking that I might be intolerant to gluten, which meant I had to give up all types of breads, salad dressings and other sauces, canned goods and so on. I tried giving up all dairy products, which can behave like glue in one's system. But all of these sacrifices came to no avail. Every day was the same anyway; slow, heavy, foggy, wracked with pain. I have heard that a severe hangover will act in much the same way, except this doesn't go away, no matter how good you are. In fact, to stay away from the source of discomfort would be to starve oneself to death.

I have lain here, in this foggy stupor, for nearly two hours now. The pain has eased but now I am stiff and oh, so cold. I will pour another hot bath. I shan't tell my doctor this. I will take my blood pressure before getting into the tub. This is the recording she will see. But what good will that do? How is she to help me if I am to manipulate my charts so that I appear to be better? I reach for my blood pressure machine, roll back my sleeve and snug it around my arm, securing the Velcro pads. I touch the ON button. It hurts to do this. I have so little blood circulating throughout this disloyal body that any delay of blood through my system renders me weak and languid. I can feel the pulses, dim at first, then increasing in intensity until my whole arm is throbbing, and I begin to feel dizzy. Just when I think I can stand it no longer, it beeps at me and releases. Ninety-two over fifty-eight with a pulse rate of ninety-six. An average reading. I will take it again after my hot bath. I will record both readings.

I sit up quickly, forgetting, my head pounding. Silly me. So forgetful. Rubbing my eyes, I make my way into the bathroom, lean over the tub, put the plug in place, turn on the hot water tap. Rarely do I need to add any cold water. I pull my hair back into a ponytail and clip my bangs back with a barrette, one of my daughter's, a green plastic barrette with a bunny rabbit on it. Bending over the sink I brush the foul taste from my mouth, then step out of my clothes, leaving them in a satisfactory heap on the linoleum floor. I gaze at my reflection in the full-length mirror. Not much has changed in twelve years. I feel shorter, more stumped over, but this is not the case. I am still five-feet-five-inches tall as I have been since I was sixteen years old. My weight has not fluctuated more than ten pounds in either direction, even during my pregnancies. My arms and shoulders are, perhaps, less meaty than they once were, and my breasts may hang a little lower, my nipples pointing downward instead of forward. My belly distends. I never did have a flat tummy. But my bottom is still shapely and round. The only distinguishable difference between this body and the one I viewed twelve years ago in another kind of mirror, is a horizontal scar along the upper edge of my pubes which has left an almost unnoticeable apron of flesh. I have heard that on the bodies of larger women, this post-surgical apron is quite grotesque, leaving them with an unsightly overhang. For this reason I am glad I am not one of those larger ladies.

It is alright to look at this body of mine. It is not alright to have to live inside it. This is the very thought that entered my mind the morning I found myself standing at the end of the dock at Pine Lake, gazing down into the water where my rippling reflection both startled and set me into a meditative state during which I first began to fall in love. How I came to be perched at the edge of the dock went something like this:

I was home again. The first heat waves of summer were just beginning to establish themselves over the prairies where they would linger in the air, motionless, but penetrating. Chirrups of crickets were the most prominent sounds this time of year. There had to have been several thousand crickets living within a hundred-foot radius of our house. At night the frogs near the pond could be heard as well, and soon the eerie cry of the coyotes would join the chorus. There is nothing quiet or hushed about the prairies during those hours of darkness. In fact, I think that there is nothing quite so satisfying and breathtaking, all at once, as that beautifully orchestrated nighttime choir.

I had moved into my bedroom full swing this time. I had no husband, no son, no best friend down the road. But my pain and tiredness were my own again and I would revel in them however I wished. The bottles of pills were discarded but since my body had become accustomed to their effects, withdrawal left me weak from insomnia and diarrhea. It passed within a couple of weeks. However, my mother, God bless her, saw to it that I had other kinds of potions and mixtures to force down my throat. She bought a state-of-the-art modern juicer and fed me carrot juice, pineapple juice, spinach juice, and so on.

In early July, my tutor handed me the keys to both her house and the lakeside cottage for me to tend while she returned to Holland for a month's visit with her younger brothers. She told me I should feel free to make use of both residences, but strongly encouraged me to take up residency at the cottage for as long as I desired or needed. So this is what I did.

The lane to her cottage had been trimmed back earlier that spring. It appeared as though my tutor had been there recently, as a week's supply of wood had been neatly stacked inside the verandah and a large pot of water had already been brought up from the spring. The first thing I did was to drag my creaky metal bed from the bedroom and set it up on wooden blocks in the kitchen area nearer the stove, where I could also cast my gaze out over the lake from my bed.

My first few days were spent wandering through the forest gathering wild flowers, which my tutor had taught me to identify during my thirteenth summer. It was surprising how many of them I could remember. I plucked fairy bells and anemones from nearer the water's edge, blue violets and pink wintergreen from the lush forest floor. I even ventured out into the fields, where I collected elephant's heads, nodding onions, even a few dandelions, and from the roadway, gathered Indian paintbrushes and common yarrow. These I arranged and placed into a ceramic pitcher and set upon the drop-leaf table in the kitchen. This was my first real home. I could do with it what I wanted. No pot roasts to brown, no potatoes to peel, no one to entertain, no appearances to be made, no one to have to speak, or explain anything to, no time constraints to follow. There was a sort of hushed reverie in going about my own business. Silence was becoming my most intimate companion.

I awoke with a start on my fourth morning from a perplexing dream in which I saw my tutor's long, splendid, naked body standing, with her arms outstretched to the heavens, on the last plank of the dock. Worship was in her stance, so graceful, reverent and powerful she stood. Both sky and water seemed to be flowing from within her body, moving through and out of her in deep, rushing torrents and returning to her in a spiraling vortex. But the dock upon which she was standing suddenly detached from the shore and began to drift out into a swirling lagoon. A group of curious onlookers had gathered on shore and were shouting obscenities, heaving stones towards her. The stones turned into bombs, which sounded like thunder. I was not on the shore watching with the crowd. Neither was I out on the lake, but somewhere above, and inside, as if in another dimension, where I could view both her exterior shell and her inner reason which had no shape, only a sorrowful and misunderstood essence. The planks, upon which she stood, rotated as they drifted, until her resplendent body was facing the belligerent crowd. There she stood, in all her defenseless, unashamed glory, those jeweled glasses sparkling and shimmering out over the water, amidst an array of fireworks. She made no attempt to cover herself, but was calmly and repeatedly whispering,

I have no need of defense.
I have no need of defense.

Daylight was just beginning to peer through the windows, casting its quiet light through myriad undefined shapes; spruce trees guarding the cottage entrance; sinuous fingers of willows reaching crookedly heavenward; and far off across the lake, the vague, dark border of the opposite shore and tree line. Melodious twittering of sparrows and larks could be heard distinctly in the morning stillness, though they had not yet begun to dart about over the lake.

Time had come to me. It could not be deferred a moment longer. Slowly I sat up, straining to see through the mist that was suspended low over the placid waters. If ever I'd heard that still, small voice about which my preacher husband had theorized so many dreary Sunday mornings, it was now, though I am sure this wasn't at all what he'd had in mind. But there it was, all the same. It was in the sweet songs of the birds perched on the boughs outside; it was in the fresh, damp, camphor aroma of pine, spruce, wild roses and last night's smoldering embers in the stove; it was in the luring mist all around, saturating the earth with new beginnings, with forgiveness. It was inside, gently pleading with me to unmask myself, step forward, surrender.

My feet found the floorboards, which were still warm from the heat of the stove and I rose, stood there beside my bed for a few moments, unsure of my next step. Then, listening, my whole body began to inch forward. The floor creaked beneath my feet. My fingers skimmed the bouquet of wild flowers. They bent humbly under my touch. It seemed as though everything had come alive during the night while I slept. But a few more paces told me that these things had always been alive. I had simply lacked the insight to perceive and understand. Twigs, spruce and pine needles felt like a lush carpet beneath by bare feet; delicate morning air clothed my bare arms and drifted right through my cotton nightgown, caressing my bare skin with its mild, velvety stillness.

The voice led me down the well-worn groove towards the waterfront and out onto the dock. My skin tightened as I pulled my nightgown over my head and let it slip to the moist planks beneath my feet. I was wide awake now, thoroughly aware of my surroundings. The whole world was holding its breath, hushed and waiting for my next move. Would it be the right one? Could I take this moment, while the world waited, to peel away the scaly sheath of worn-out flesh that was holding me in its unmerciful clutches? Could I allow myself to lower my banner of pain, and the fear of that pain? Could I learn to love my pain, to mold it like clay, shape it into something beautiful, something worthy of my love?

I stepped to the edge. The water looked black, threatening. Whatever lay beneath its surface I could not know from above.

Then I saw it. I saw her - distorted, rippling, fluid, capable of shape-changing, yet still one, unified reflection. I saw the figure of another woman down there; a woman whose naked form made me think of a fruit tree during harvest, ripe and succulent and tender; a woman without pain, without fear or limitations. She spoke to me. It was the voice inside, but I needed to be nearer for I could not hear her.

I remember exactly how it felt, plunging into the lake that early July morning, how the water seemed to open up and embrace me, hugging my tired body in its stimulating, nourishing coolness. I came up through the water, breaking the surface, gasping from the shock, my whole body tingling. I wanted to shout, or laugh, but not even a single peep came from within. I heard her voice though, clear and undeniable. And this is what she whispered,

Welcome home.

I had lived without spoken words or human contact for four days. As I hoisted myself up onto the planks of the dock I realized that audible words were no longer necessary. Communication could be carried on without spoken language. To be silent also meant preserving vital breath which could be utilized in more efficient, substantive ways. I do not think that I consciously took a vow of silence that morning. Silence found me.

Of course I would never share these intimate moments, these memories I have, with anyone. People think me daft enough without knowing of my inner musings, my secret, sacramental wanderings. But I cannot help myself. The body I have been given to live inside is the only one I've got. It hurts, it cries out in agony. Sometimes I think it betrays me, so unwieldy and disagreeable it is. But its constant pain has unveiled another realm. A realm of beauty, where the ready and supple fruit has broken, exposing its seed to both sun and rain, bringing life and understanding to all things. Without my pain I would see only the surface, the plain exterior where true, living color does not exist. Without my pain I would not know the experience of pleasure. Without my pain I would be an empty vessel. My body, this shell of anguish that encloses my soul, has been my path towards love.

A funny thing happened not too many days after that baptism. I was sitting on shore, my knees tucked up to my chest, my arms folded across my knees. I was watching the boaters, the skiers, the fishers, for the lake was a flurry of activity on that sweltering hot summer day. I had no thoughts really, no plans, and certainly no action, when along the shoreline glided a green fiberglass canoe. Its occupant, clad in khaki shorts and tank top, waved to me as he paddled by. He was tall and lithesome, wearing a steady, sanguine expression on his silky-smooth face. I watched his hands methodically lifting and plunging the paddle in regular circular motions. They were strong, those hands. Strong and sturdy, but with an easy, comfortable grip.

I smiled when he turned and paddled back the other way, and laughed to myself when back he came a third time and, after disappearing around the embankment, a fourth time, and a fifth. Even when I waved him to shore and gestured that he join me, I could not speak aloud. He spoke very loudly to me, close to my face, and exaggerated his enunciations, thinking I was deaf and mute. And I felt no inclination to explain, not even with paper and pen. This must have been alright with him because he came back the following day and then the next, and the day after that.

Eventually I married him.

shshshshshshshshshshsh

Even now I must be silent sometimes. Silence is a language far more eloquent and lasting than any spoken word the history of civilization has ever dreamt. I do not choose when to be silent or when to speak. Silence chooses me. Sometimes it just becomes necessary to listen to my thoughts without the interference or diversion of sound. My thoughts are birds, which cannot fly in the confines of a cage. They crave solitude and space, and become tangled in the crowd of too many words.

My husband pats my bottom a lot when I go inside myself like this. He says he understands. He doesn't, of course, and I wouldn't want him to. He would be frightened and horribly lonely inside the stillness of my mind. He is a more social being, a man of beautiful words, simple words at which I sometimes have to laugh because they are so marvelously simple. Buffalo roam inside his mind. Buffalo and deer and antelope. He has no cognizance of a discouraging word.

How did I get from there to here? Twelve years have sifted through my fingers and all my musings and wonderings can't bring them back. I've seen ninety-year-old men and women, who have lived far longer and far greater lives, brood less about their fading lives than I do. How did I get to be thirty-five when last time I checked I was only twenty-three and a new mother again? I've heard that at the moment of death a person's whole life flashes before his or her eyes. I would like to think that my brooding, my constant backlash of memories and contemplations, is an indication that the end is nearing. But I shouldn't be so fortunate. I have envied those terminally ill, those in hospital beds doped up on morphine, passing their final moments away in an oblivious stupor. Death is a blessing. But I have been cursed with living. It goes on and on and on. I'm not allowed to just quit. Quitting isn't socially acceptable.

He didn't require anything of me, my angel husband. But I didn't do nothing. I made more babies. I cannot, for the life of me, understand why I did this except that it seemed to be all the rage at the time. People got married, made babies, struggled with bills, bought a house, then struggled with bigger bills. They smelled like a diaper pale. Their children outgrew diapers, started school, got into trouble and were bailed out of jail. Then they smelled like whiskey. Wives got fat and blabby. Husbands went bald and filled a groove on the couch. Eventually the children grew up and got married too and the cycle repeated itself.

I haven't been terribly strict about following these rules. For instance, I didn't join the baby-sitting pool. I never went anywhere that I couldn't take my kids. During those early years of marriage I believed in the socialist ideal of community. My husband's mother still lived nearby, in Innisfail, where she had lived her entire life. Two brothers and a sister were in Sundre, and the youngest sister, only a ten-minute drive from here. We were all marrying and making babies around the same time. A baby boy first, then a baby girl, then two more girls and then a boy and two more on the way. I thought we could all help one another. I thought that's what families did.

I was wrong.

Very, very wrong.

But I still made the best pot roasts, apple pies and

homemade ice cream. After setting the feast out on our eight-foot-long table, which my husband had built to accommodate his large family, I would vanish from the scene, go away somewhere and lie down where my thoughts would not be crowded by obligatory chitchat. They didn't know I was within earshot range, lying on the trampoline beneath the deck, stretching out my aching knees.

Well she's gone and disappeared again, as usual. Thinks she's too high and mighty for the rest of us. is what spewed from the blabby mouth of one of these family members whose name I needn't divulge. *Well, at least I didn't throw my child away, neither have I been divorced, and at least I take my children to Sunday school. My family doesn't have to put up with a depressed wife and mother who pretends to be tired and anorexic and parades around in the nude to show it off.*

Well I think she's lonely, is what the other mused, in a measly attempt to defend my tendency towards aloofness. *I think she's just not used to this, being an only child and all. Probably she was babied a lot.*

Well sooner or later she has to grow up and start taking some responsibility. I can't understand why our brother married her, or why he stays with her.

Maybe he thinks nobody else would love her.

Or maybe he stays because of the kids.

I watched a talk show the other day about psychosomatics - people who think they have pain but there's absolutely nothing the matter with them except that they believe they're in pain. It's not right, you know. He ought to do something about it instead of letting her get away with it all the time. Can you imagine just dumping your own child like that, as if it doesn't even exist? There's got to be something wrong upstairs.

Of course it hurt. Did she think I wanted to leave my child behind? My eldest offspring with the shadowy dark eyes, raven hair and rotund features patterned after his handsome father's? What did they know of letting go of your own flesh and blood, a child to whom you gave birth, lent life, and nursed three-hundred-and-sixty-five nights in a row? What did they know of pain and tiredness? What did they know of responsibility?

I wanted my son to love me. I wanted him to be my best friend. I called my ex-sister-in-law weekly for awhile to see how my son was getting along. But she only provided me with vague, quasi-information.

Oh he's fine, she would say. Or if I wanted to talk to him, hear him gurgle or babble over the phone, she would tell me, *he's sleeping right now*, or *he's busy playing outside with his cousin right now. Why don't you call back later?* Or she would put him on the phone and I would say,

Hi, Baby, do you know who this is? And then my sister-in-law would nab the phone back and say,

Well, we don't want to run up your phone bill or tie up the phone line for too long. Call again. Click.

They did send pictures, though, when I asked. My son was, indeed, a beautiful little boy. The photos were full of action. He would be tricycling down the driveway, or climbing their white picket fence or shooting the neighbor kid with his plastic dart gun. They had managed to capture a snapshot of him sleeping, in a child's bed, tangled in a boyish quilt of colorful trucks and motorcycles. His long eyelashes curled into a quarter-moon and the pillow appeared moist beneath his open mouth. I ran my fingertips along the surface of the photo and tried to remember what his creamy-smooth baby skin felt like; hot and moist sometimes, when he'd had a fever; soft and silky during the night when he'd been sleeping. I remembered his baby fingers curling around mine, grasping them with all his baby might; I remembered the imprint of his tiny feet in plaster when he was five days old and how I used to nuzzle my nose up against his fuzzy, soft head, breathing in that pure, subtle, baby fragrance, the delicate newness, ultimate innocence.

But he didn't want me. He screamed at me, threw things at me, bit me with those miniature white teeth of his, ran away from me. He was happy in his new home. And that's what I wanted most of all. I wanted my son to grow up happy.

Maybe one day he will visit me. He will be thickset and barrel-chested like his preacher father. His black hair will be thick and wavy. He will have to keep it cut short, otherwise it would grow upward and outward and get away on him. He will have inflexible, rubbery ears that grow red in the slightest breeze. He will have been shaving since he was fourteen years old. His voice will be strong but melodious and smooth. The words that he speaks will be spoken with passion and sincerity. He will not be unkind, but will stand his ground. He will be firm and resolute.

Perhaps when I am old my eldest son will look after me. He will pat my withered, peppery hands and say,
Oh, Mother.
Will he ever call me Mother? Will he even know he has a mother?

I don't speak of him much. Not out loud. That certain relation of mine can say what she wants. How would she feel if she'd had to lose a son? Has she ever even asked me?

My second son was so unlike my first that I wondered if there had been a baby exchange day at the hospital to which I hadn't been invited. He was fair-skinned and tiny, with a button nose, and freckled like Wilma. He never screeched at me the way my first son had. He never even cried. He merely whimpered when he was hungry and made no noise at all when his diaper needed changing. He was so quiet that I would wake with a start at night. The lack of crying is what would wake me, the noiselessness coming from his crib. Candid blue eyes would watch my every move, as though he were studying me to memorize the things that made me happy or what made me sorrowful. When he learned to walk, he would follow me around, tugging gently, almost imperceptibly, at my pant legs. At night, sometimes, I would wake and there he would be, standing by our bed, as quiet and motionless as the stuffed toys lining his bedroom walls.

Ninga, is what he would say in a petite, facile voice. *Ninga?*

But during my next pregnancy my body weight plummeted to a slight one-hundred-ten pounds. I lived in a perpetual haze of dizzying nausea. Everything I ate tasted like charred rubber and landed with a thud in my stomach. Sometimes it would come back out, without warning. We would be having dinner around my husband's grand family table and I would be forking a bite of food into my mouth, but instead, food would come out of my mouth. Naturally, my in-laws were repelled at this latest stunt, but soon grew used to it. I would listen, from my bed in the other room, to the nattering about these attention-seeking antics of mine.

Whatever does she think she's doing having another child anyway? spat the one. *She can't even handle the ones she's got.*

Well it's really none of our business, the other would volunteer in a possible attempt at diffusing the allegations.

Doesn't our brother know that he'll be raising those kids all by himself? How is he supposed to raise kids and run after her every whim and fancy?

My daughter slid into this world while my husband and the doctor were down the corridor in the cafeteria filling their plates and bellies on a Chinese buffet. They barely made it back in time for my husband to cut the chord and wipe the goo out of his daughter's bleary eyes. She didn't look anything like my other two children, and totally unlike anyone on either side of the family. She was long in the body, her toes were joined together with bridges of pink skin, webbed like duck's feet, and she had a peach-like, downy fuzz all over her tiny, wriggling body.

Oh, she's beautiful! my husband exclaimed through his tears. *She looks just like you, Honey.* Of course, my husband is half-blind and everything he lays eyes on is beautiful to him. What I wouldn't give to have his vision.

There was a mirror on the wall opposite the birthing bed. Afterwards, when my daughter had been bundled in flannel blankets and the nurse was massaging my sore belly to encourage remnants of afterbirth and fluids to drain, I caught a glimpse of my reflection in that mirror and only then remembered that I had witnessed the horror and holiness of my daughter's birth.

This is what I saw:

A woman's face twisting into alien-like contortions, in apparent excruciating pain; sorrowful, imploring eyes gazing back at me, wordlessly pleading for a single moment of relief; rocking like a pendulum, as though the rocking would lull her away from the awful, wrenching agony; others, other humans, one gripping the alien woman's hand, blue-veined, purple with clenching, another one with a hand on the desperate woman's swollen belly, easing, propelling the swelling downward and outward; another one near the end of the bed, looking down, his hands outstretched in a sort of welcoming pose; a hole, a black hole growing larger, wider, ripping, bleeding; grotesque, oozing red, creamy fluid; a protrusion in the black hole, a slimy outgrowth, twisting, pushing its way through; blackness, then nothing, then blinding lights; then again the protrusion forcing its way out; then a gush of fluids, tiny arms and legs flailing in a sticky creamy-white mess like cottage cheese and mayonnaise; the woman, wide-eyed, amazed, exhausted; and a satiny-smooth rope, incredible deep mauve-blue, pulsating purple, winding around and around. There was no sound at all. None. Not even silence.

My mother arrived bearing her latest craze.

Barley Green. It cures any ailment. Try it and see. It's not so bad really, once you get used to it. I find it quite refreshing in the morning.

It was horrible of course, worse than her brewer's yeast conglomerations. It tasted like the contents of a barn. But I gulped it down anyway. It put a satisfied glow onto her cheeks to watch me swallow that green slime.

She cuddled and cooed over my downy daughter.

I suppose I did everything I should have done. I took my son to hockey practice even though most evenings I could barely stumble through the arena, my legs and feet deadweights, plunking heavily across the concrete floor. The other mothers would bring horns and bells and they would cheer, applaud and screech at the top of their lungs, shaking those god-awful bells and blowing ear-numbing horns. When my son scored I didn't leap up and shout or hop about on the bleachers. I sat there huddling, shivering, apart from the other bellering mothers, and cried. I don't know why I cried. I can't explain some of these emotions and why they fly sporadically about the way they do. Often they don't match the occasion at all.

Like this:

When one of my sister-in-law's elderly grandmothers died, I giggled. I didn't mean to. Giggling just seemed the thing to do. In my mind, giggling was much more appropriate than tears, remorse or grief. The old lady, who was at least a century old, was propped up in her casket, clearly a misfit amidst the ruffles, the lacy, virgin-white pillows. She was little more than a clothed skeleton, wasted and tiny, her skin pasty and rouged with make-up. She looked like a ghoulish clown, a Halloween costume without a body in it. So I giggled. From behind, it may have appeared as though I had been stricken with grief, my shoulders were shaking so. But oh, the looks of exaggerated scorn thrown in my direction. If Wilma had been there, we would have had to restrain ourselves from dashing up there and poking the dead old lady, then scurrying away before the consequences caught up with us.

This is what I mean about displaying a mismatch of emotion and event. In my younger days, my father and I used to play a matching game called Memory. The game consisted of about two dozen pairs of cards. One side was a continuous pattern, and on the other side was a picture of some animal, bird or fish. When they were all flipped over with the pattern side up, the game began. You could flip over only two cards. If they were a matching pair, you got another turn and whoever ended up with the most matching pairs won the game. But I had some difficulty with this. The baby bear and the baby rabbit looked the same to me. So did the elephant and the ostrich.

I don't mean to be such a social misfit. My husband doesn't seem to mind. It doesn't matter to him what I do or say. His love for me is unchanging, unconditional. He would run ahead of me and pick the pebbles from my path if he could. But he can't because the pebbles are inside of me. A ton of them.

He has been good to me, my husband. He is patient and kind and generous to a fault, if that is possible. There is nothing he wouldn't do for me to make my life more comfortable, or at the very least, less uncomfortable.

Once I wanted to play the piano. I thought that if I could create a soundtrack to back up my dull, musicless life it would be more bearable, interesting even. He didn't buy me any old piano. He bought me a Yamaha L106, with a glossy black finish that now stands tall and stately in the corner gathering dust. It is also useful for the gaudy lamp that my kind-hearted mother-in-law picked up at a flea market, thinking it would be lovely set upon my piano. I learned to play chopsticks and the first three measures of Fur Elise. By the fourth measure my fingers got all jammed up and piled on each other.

After the piano phase petered out, I thought I would like to do pottery. It looked so easy and elegant on television. Therapeutic. Heavenly. A lump of clay was thrown onto a whirring wheel. Muddy water was dribbled over the lump from a sponge. Then goopy hands were placed around it. Within mere seconds it had been miraculously transformed from a shapeless lump into a slender, shapely vase. I was most impressed with the potter himself, however, who wore an apron which read, *throw naked,* across the front and was splattered with clay. There were also patches of dried clay clinging to the man's face and all the way up his arms. Clay was also matted in the hair on his bare legs and oozed between his toes, for his trousers were rolled up to his calves and he wore leather sandals on his feet. The shop, in which he muddied himself, was strewn with strange and lovely shapes of all sizes. There were no bright colors, only mat earth tones, much like Wilma's skin. Mud was everywhere. How remarkable! How daring and utterly gratifying to be able to smear mud about like that and not be compelled, by some insane sense of obligation, to clean it up! This was how I wanted to be. Reckless, unrestrained, unabashedly creative.

So my husband bought me a wheel, and not just any old wheel. He bought me a Shimpo-top-of-the-line, and ten boxes of clay, most of which are now molding in a corner of the garage. My fingers seemed to lack the agility and strength needed to massage the clay into a workable lump, and after only one session, my hands shriveled up from dryness and began to crack and bleed. It hurt.

> *So many things to do and be,*
> *whether we are he or she.*

Sometimes I think I would like to write. Reading is wonderful, gathering and absorbing radical ideas, or sometimes just plain ordinary ideas that I haven't yet considered. But sometimes I think I would like to write. Such a silly notion poofs off into space the moment it is conceived however. Whatever would I have to write about? My life is a long series of nothing. What have I behind me but drudgery? What is there in my present everyday life that would be worth telling?

And what is before me but a dull replay of the past and present? I would have to delve into the realm of science fiction, something totally out of this world, but then there is the problem of creation. Creativity requires focus and I have the focusing capacity of a toothpick. I have spoken with Peggy about this of course. She tells me that I am mistaken.

Everybody has a story to tell. A well told story is not in the story itself, is what she tells me, *but rather, in its telling.*

If Peggy were alive today I would want to meet her. I would want more than to meet her. I would want to be her friend. I would follow her around like a puppy licking and nipping at her ankles, begging for attention. She would eventually have to kick me away and shout at me to go home. She would have to chase me away with a stick.

No, I wouldn't, says Peggy.

I do not tell my husband about this. I am afraid he would rush out and purchase a computer for me with all the latest in writing programs and he would encourage me and say things like,

What have you written today? or, *How's my little writer doing?* or, *How's the story coming?* and I would have nothing to report.

So I don't really allow myself to want much anymore because the disappointment of failure is harder to bear than the frustration of wanting to try. So I just leave it alone now - all those unmet desires, the things I wanted to do, places I wanted to go, feelings I wanted to have. It is too much like trying to look through a boarded up window. I don't bother looking anymore. I know what's there, and what isn't.

This is alright though, too. This is my life. I have been given very few tools with which to chisel away at this life, but I have tried to do my maker justice with what I have. What else can I do? I cannot buy comfort and ease from someone else. I cannot even steal it. And no one can give it to me, though my husband, the angel, does try. He tries to understand, but how could he, really? To thoroughly understand, to be able to truly empathize, one must feel what the other person feels and I do not wish my husband to feel what I feel. He would die. He would just give up and die. Most people would, I think. Whatever compels me to remain standing, I haven't quite figured out, though not for lack of trying.

He views me as some sort of rare exotic flower that doesn't require a great deal of attention. Just admiration. He looks at me and bends his head side to side, flapping those puppy eyelashes. He touches me and pats me and constantly asks if there is anything he can do for me. There never is. Sometimes he says this to me,

Shall I compare thee to a summer's day? Thou art more lovely and more temperate. Although he has no idea where this quote originated, hearing it makes me very proud of him for trying.

He is steady and true. I ask myself everyday if I am truly deserving of his love and devotion. I ask myself how I got to be thirty-five years old when just a moment ago I was becoming his bride. He has been faithful to me all these years in every way. And I have been faithful to my beloved in every way.

Except one.

shshshshshshshshshsh

It didn't last long, that brief interlude I had with the cowpoke over at the edge of town some years ago. He lived in an Airstream bus in the middle of a fenced twenty-acre pasture, two horses, two geese and a cow. I don't know that I can, or want to, recall his name. It was something simple and shortened, like Joe, or Pete, or Art. A name that could easily have been absorbed by greater, more significant memories.

I had failed at creating a fantastic piece of musicianship and a house full of clay pots and mud. I thought I could try something out of the ordinary, something out of My ordinary. A guest of Oprah Winfrey purported once, that all marriages are one hundred percent subject to infidelity. So in this regard, there was nothing extraordinary about it. I guess it was pleasure I was after, not even pleasure. Relief would have sufficed. Even numbness would have been enough.

He said he would take me away from here and I thought that if I could just get away from some of these nattery people and their accusations, away from my busy children even, if I could rest, no responsibilities to weigh me down, I could get better. Maybe not completely, but enough to function.

I only wanted to be made love to without having to exert a lot of uncomfortable effort. I wanted to feel another human body beside mine, or on top of mine, or under mine. A human body more my size. A body that could move with me without being too heavy or obtrusive. Perhaps angels are not endowed with such carnal knowledge, that very earthy animal instinct from which we all suffer.

When I was certain that my transgression had come to an end, I explained it to my husband, not in detail of course, but with enough particulars that he would not be misled into thinking that it was nothing. It wasn't nothing. It was wonderful. Beautiful at the time. Now I wonder how I could have allowed that completely cragged, non-committal man to monopolize my thoughts the way he did so that I would wait anxiously every day for his phone call.

My emotional state would be governed by his presence, or lack of presence; his voice on the phone, his voice and hands imprinted into my supple, impressionable mind; the memories of his lips caressing my neck; the smell of him, musky, unwashed; the sweet, clingy scent of chewing tobacco on his breath; the sensuous feel of thick, mossy hair spread out over his face, his chest, his abdomen, and the curl of lint that found its way into his navel after a hard day's work. He looked and felt like the muscular, gray bark of a gnarled old elm. If we did not see one another or speak for a couple of days I would feel rejected, unworthy again, alone in my pain, the vulturous world circling about me waiting for a weak moment in which to attack.

When we were together I wanted to breathe him in. I felt that if I could absorb the essence of him into my lungs, it would spread through my entire being, through every cell, and he would remain in there forever. Some people take pictures. Some people write it down. Some try to remember with their minds' eye. Our olfactory system is more closely linked to the emotion site in our brains than any of our other senses. This is why, when we catch a whiff of a certain peculiar scent, we are suddenly carted away to Grandmother's kitchen, or reminded of blackberries and bee stings, the boot room of the elementary school building, and so on, and these memories trigger certain emotions to match the event.

I thought I could contain him in my memory this way,

alive, moveable, palpable. I would sometimes envelop myself in one of his unwashed shirts. I would wrap it around my shoulders, my neck, sink my nose into its soft, male fragrance, close my eyes, drinking in his essence with an unyielding urgency as though I were parched and might die of thirst if I did not gulp it down fast enough.

I did not want my passion to overrun my reason for I knew that this was exactly what was happening to me but I was powerless to resist. I said this aloud on his bed, tangled in his blankets and sheets, wrapped in his shirt and in his arms. My fingers were tracing the fine contours of his whiskered face. He had the features of one descended from the gods. A fine, triangular nose, nostrils flared only a little; sculptured cheekbones, weathered with rugged elegance; and the lines around his eyes and upon his brow spoke of both merriment and pain through many years of arduous outdoor labor.

If I'd wanted to, I felt it would have been possible to smooth out those wrinkles, stretch his skin back into its rudimentary youthful form and I would have been able to behold him as a boy, fresh and alive with innocent anticipation; as a young man, sleek and muscled, imbued with insatiable passion and vigor; I could have watched him age, viewed every event of his life as it unfolded, taken note of every line, tear and scar as it appeared, spreading over his face like rivers on a map; I would have seen this marvelous creation being sculpted before my eyes, under my fingertips, my lips. I would have known exactly what had carved him into the beautiful creature he had become. But I didn't want to do that. I only wanted now, the moment. But I wanted that moment to last into infinity.

When I touched him in this way, he would close his eyes, his mouth, and his breathing would slow. It would seem as if he was immersed in a dream or deep meditative state, except for slow, barely audible murmurs and sighs. I must have touched or soothed something inside him, something that made him pause in his busy lifestyle to accept my caresses. Could he have known that I was taking of him more than he was willing to give? I could accuse myself of thievery, but he'll never know just what I took from him. He doesn't miss it in the least. He doesn't know that a great chunk of him is irreplaceably lost to him.

This is what I heard myself saying in his bed, our limbs, like the branches of that great elm, entangled together, becoming one in their reach for the heavens,

Your soul is oftentimes a battlefield, upon which your reason and your judgment wage war against your passion and your appetite.

A low soft moan came from somewhere inside him. My fingers were following the curves of his ears. There were no creases on his earlobes, which meant he had good circulation, his heart was strong. He had a long life yet ahead of him. His eyes didn't open when he muttered, smiling,

That's what I like about you. For any occasion, you can just come up with a quote, or a bit of poetry. You intrigue me, the way your mind works.

He stumbled on the word, *intrigue*, as though unsure of its use in the sentence, not wishing to appear unlearned.

You can be so quiet. Nobody knows what you're thinking. We all notice that. But now that I know you, it makes me wonder even more. I think about you all the time, every hour, every minute. I wonder where you are, what you're doing, what you're reading. Mostly I wonder what you're thinking, and why. When we're together, you say so little. But when you do talk, you say something totally unexpected and I have to think about it for awhile before I understand. Sometimes I don't really understand at all but I still like to hear your voice. I do like to hear you talk.

I had my own fascinations, my own special objects of intrigue. My fingers were running themselves over the creases of his forehead, through his mass of spiraling hair that wound up into wiry curls behind his ears. At times like these, my hands were a maze of minds of their own. They would open and close, grasping bunches of hair, drawing them closer to my face, brushing my cheeks, my neck, with their bristly softness.

But I only speak when I run out of things to think about, is what I replied in a whisper.

This was quite true. To speak aloud meant to deplete my precious stores of oxygen, thus draining my sensitive physical form of its energy. Besides, in moments such as this, I didn't feel words were necessary, and were, in fact, intrusive.

To love him, to explore his regions unknown to me, to bask in his vital energy, indulge in a luxury so foreign to me, and allow myself to be carried away without effort, without thought, without pain, was a means of worship, in much the same way as the moment of baptism in my tutor's lake. This was my experience. Like my pain and unremitting fatigue, no one could experience this for me. No one else could possibly even begin to perceive the depth, the height and breadth of this, my spiritual quest. This was my way of seeking justice, equilibrium, in an otherwise world of imbalance. I felt almost at eye level to the gods, and my presence here was beyond acceptable, favored, honored. Here was the intermingling, the marriage, of joy and sorrow.

Wise men say nothing in dangerous times.

Is this a dangerous time?

Without question. You are outside the boundaries of my safety net. You are in a position to unravel my carefully wound-up soul. With you I rock the edge of sanity.

Don't you mean insanity?

No, I mean complete and utter sanity.

Can't you speak my language for once?

I think I love you, is how I answered him.

I am not attempting to justify my actions in any way. I am simply remembering it the way it was. It is not as though my life was wanting. My life was full, brimming, running over with busyness. The tediousness of tending to my children, dodging the spears of my in-laws, caring for my angel. Perhaps, in a way, this brief, beautiful interlude, was just that - an interlude, a pause, a break in space-time from the agony of every day living.

In retrospect I wonder how I could have managed the added energy it took to fit all of those heightened emotions into my already crowded right hemisphere. And where did I unearth the physical strength needed to find myself in his company, whether it was just a walk, grasping hands, up river, stepping from stone to stone, laughing like giddy children, or a five hour exploration of each others' tingling, burning bodies. There was no work involved, only pleasure. I suspect that the reason I recall so little physical pain during this time, is because most often, we were horizontal, rolling together, entwined in the throes of passion, or lying side by side, resting. At what other time in my daily life did I stop just to rest, while all thoughts of discomfort and distress were pushed aside by pure pleasure, however indulgent it may have been? Not once. Not ever.

When are you going to pack up your pajamas and come live with me? You could live with me couldn't you? is what he asked me, pulling a t-shirt over his tousled head.

Yes. Yes, of course I could, is how I responded, bringing his worn flannel shirt closer to my face, breathing in the greasy-sweet traces of his workday.

And this, also, was true. I could live with just about anybody. I could live with King Kong or Rumplestiltskin if I had to. And I would be committed and fair. I would aim to please.

This is how it came about that I began to try in earnest to explain to him what he was getting into, the sort of life he would have with me in his house, in his bed, all around him, permeating his every thought and move, with or without my actual physical presence. I wanted him to understand that, although I could be an intelligent, obliging amusement and would love him with all of my meager might, keeping me would be a high maintenance project for which he might not quite be prepared.

I know you get tired sometimes, is how he tried to assure us both after I'd brought up the dismal subject of my evasive

116

health. But I was disappointed with this very understated, incomplete summary, which implied a serious deficit in comprehension.

Tired, I said slowly, enunciating my words with purposeful precision, *is something you are after a very hard day's work. I do not get tired. Tired is something I felt about twenty-five years ago. Tired is only the very tip of the iceberg. Underneath, for miles and miles down, is total exhaustion. More than exhaustion. Painful exhaustion, to the point where you wish you could stop breathing. You wish it could end. You think about making it end. But you're too exhausted to try anything.*

Hey now, don't go talking like that. That's no good.

No, you must try to understand this. I am not unhappy. This is my life. This is how I live. Every day. Every night. I can't eat. I can't sleep. I can't be awake. My heart pounds inside me, sometimes it threatens to explode. Sometimes I feel so weak and ill that all I can do is crumple up on the floor and wait. Wait for it to stop. But it doesn't stop. Only when I'm with you do I feel okay. And that's because all we ever do is lie here.

When you're with me, you'll be better. See, you said so yourself. You'll get your strength back in no time at all. So go pack up your jammies and come live with me.

I shook him. I pounded on his shoulders, took his beautiful, innocent face into my hands, looked into his uncomprehending, ashy-blue eyes.

You're not listening! This is real! This is what I've been trying to tell you, show you. How can you think you'll make me better? Do you think you've got some magical potion that no doctor in the world has yet been able to give me, or anybody else inflicted with this horrible illness? What makes you think you'll be the one? What makes you so sure?

I just know, that's how.

Please - please try to understand. Can't you understand?

I'm trying to. All I know is that I'm happy when you're with me. And I think that you are too. You won't have to do

117

anything. I'll take care of you. I want to do that. I know you're fragile. He grabbed my waist, his hands edging up under my heavy sweater, his fingers running over my scanty ribcage. *And I want you to do something for me.* The silver ring he wore on the fourth finger of his right hand felt cold and hard against my skin. *This here,* he said, grasping both of my shoulder blades, *is too thin. I want you to put on some weight.*

Sure, is all I could say. He didn't understand. How could I expect him to? How could I expect that of anyone? I looked well, didn't I? Isn't that what was said? My skin, though it was often afflicted with unexplainable blistery rashes that kept me awake at night for the unrelievable itching, was usually tinted with just the right pigment; my eyes were the same hazy gray-blue they had always been, never red or glassy or peaked; I was not at all emaciated, and in fact, wore an apron of flesh around my belly and healthy bulges on my thighs. I did not appear to be ill in the least. The only manifestation of any malady was behind my skin, deep inside my muscles and bones, on the inside of each cell membrane, where it ripped through my body with unforgiving heaviness and often searing spasms.

Pain is only real when someone else believes that your pain is real. Otherwise, if no one believes in your pain, it is craziness, something you have contrived in your mind, an hallucination.

I sighed. What else was there to do or say?

I bent my head towards his chest, pressing my forehead against the regular pattering of his heartbeat. It made me think of a wind-up clock I'd had as a child. It had a plastic sphere in the center, which rotated with each tick-tock. On the sphere were glow-in-the-dark comets and stars. Lying there in my attic bedroom each night, I used to watch those heavenly bodies go round and round, luring me to sleep with their comforting, regular steadiness. Inside the cavity of his chest I felt and heard the same rhythmic clockwork pulsing steadily, immutably onward. And once again, I was on the outside, looking and listening in, eavesdropping on an elusive and forbidden fantasy. I was twirling around in the event horizon, forever sinking, never disappearing, always out of reach.

Listen to me. I want you to be with me. I love you. Very much. Very, very much. And I know you feel the same way about me. I like the way you are. I like the way you dress. I like how you make me think. I love those things about you, and if we love each other, what else matters?

After awhile, shortly after that ineffectual discussion about the consequences my health might have on our relationship, he quit coming around as much. First, it was a week, then two, then a month between our encounters. Each time he told me, with emotional surety to the point of actual tears, that he loved me. But I should have known, right from the beginning, because he said these kinds of things to me:

I would never hurt you. I'll never lie to you. Why would I lie to you? I'll wait for you, as long as it takes. I won't leave here without you. I want you to be with me.

I told myself then, that it was funny he didn't say, *I want to be with you*, but the more egocentric version, *I want YOU to be with ME.*

He also said,

I shouldn't be doing this. A married woman. And your husband is such a good guy. I told myself I would never ever do this. But I just can't help myself. I have to.

It was mid autumn, like it is now, the sun extraordinarily brilliant and low in the horizon; burnished golden leaves scarcely fluttering in the temperate breeze. The earth was, once again, growing sleepy, preparing for its downy blanket of fallen leaves, dusty foliage, then snow, beneath which it would rejuvenate itself for another infinite cycle of seasons.

It must have been around ten o'clock a.m. when I finally dragged myself from my bed, struggled into a pair of rubber boots, tossed a sweater over my pajamas and headed out into that balmy morning. I took a deep breath and clambered up the ladder into the loft of the barn where I would heave a bale of hay down to the horses, whose store of grass had dwindled to almost nothing during the last week.   Our three horses had congregated at the base of the barn door and didn't budge when sections of hay fell out of the loft on top of them. They merely began chewing contentedly, rustling through their dusty breakfast for the best pickings.

My mind was twirling with its usual melancholy meditations of my lover, even though I had been attempting to subdue them during the last few weeks with a mind-over-matter approach, as I had felt his all-encompassing presence slipping through my jaded fingers. What right had I to even wish for his sustaining affection? What could I offer him that he couldn't find more abundantly elsewhere? I had entertained notions about leaving my husband and my children to go be with him, but reality dictated that I should stay right where I was and let him go on with his life without me to inconvenience him any more than I already had.

I think what I really wanted was just to be alone.

This is what I was thinking the moment his black-capped head appeared above the ladder. He was gazing at me with a dejected, almost vanquished, strain in his unblinking blue eyes. I wanted to run to him. I wanted to step right inside him, curl up in some out-of-the-way corner of his soul. I would be a shadow inside him, not even requiring space in which to breathe. I would meld into his essence. I would be his vital breath.

My bounty is as boundless as the sea;
 my love is as deep.
The more I give to you,
 the more I have;
 for both are infinite.

I did not quote this aloud, but whispered it deep inside my own disconsolate soul. I had no words or thoughts of my own with which to augment that moment, seeing him there amidst the dusty scent of hay, horse and cobwebs, the two of us consumed by our own finite world of possibilities.

He eased himself up onto the floorboards, dusted off his hands, then reached for me, tugging gently, imploringly, at the edge of my pajama top. No audible words were exchanged. We knelt there together midst the dry, cobwebbed beams and prickly mounds of loose hay, in a kind of reverent plea, the horses munching and rustling beneath us. I thought I saw a tear escape his sorrowful eyes, but was mistaken. The tear had come from my own eye.

I just thought I'd drop by, is what he said to me after some time had elapsed. *But I've got to get going. I'll see you later.*

I thought of Wilma, wondered if she had a barn in which to sit and muse about the goings on of the world as we had when we were young and carefree. I thought of our games of hide-and-seek, how much we giggled, giving ourselves away, unable to keep silent or still in that great, childhood cathedral full of wonderful hiding places. But when the game was over, we'd both had to go home.

The game appeared to be over. Time to go home.

It wasn't his fault. He was just an ordinary man with ordinary ambition and ordinary understanding. Was I expecting too much when I wanted him to understand, believe and accept me? I would like to think that our gradual parting was due to an awakening, on his part, of an innate sense of nobility that forbade him to tread on another man's territory. I would like to believe that he had meant every one of those beautiful words that flowed from his beautiful lips and that, by reason of virtue, he had begun to comprehend that I was not an ordinary woman, and that, perhaps, my husband was, after-all, the better man for the job. I would like to believe that he did, and does, indeed, love me in some quiet, unassuming way and that is why he quit pestering me to pack up my jammies and unpack them in his bureau drawer.

It began in the winter, just before Christmas, and persisted throughout the spring, summer and into the fall. Then it seemed to wander off, perhaps, I hoped, just to find a den in which to hibernate. I waited through the winter for it to re-emerge and in the spring, made a semi-conscious effort to awaken what seemed to have just fallen asleep. But no amount of rousing, hinting, placing myself in his path could bring it back. I could have gone to him, openly, pressing my desires, my hopes, upon his pliable will. But we could not have concealed our secret affiliation for much longer anyway. I would have wanted to shout it to the world, so grand, lovely and almost well, I felt by his side. What choice did I have but to let it go before it degenerated into an all or nothing policy? It had served its purpose, had provided me with intense relief, given me a reason to plow myself through each painful day and turbulent night.

Pleasure is a powerful opiate.

My husband was pushing back the cuticles of his fingernails with the thumbnail of the other hand while I told him this. I did not bother to tell him how powerful the liaison had been, how much deeper and further in it had gone than a simple infatuation, that it had expanded my heart until it had nearly imploded in upon itself. When I ceased talking, he said, without looking up,

So it's all over with now, is it?

I nodded, but he wasn't looking at me so I said, *Yes.* Then he looked over at me with great tenderness, and a bit of sadness, and said with a slight nod,

Well then, I guess that's that. He then got up, kissed me on the cheek, patted my bottom and said, *I'm going out to feed the horses. Want to come?*

Well then, I guess that's that. Those are the exact words

he'd used once when I'd forgotten to latch the rabbit cage and they'd all scampered away during the night. *Well then, I guess that's that.*

When he dies, that beautiful, unforgettable man that captured my whole essence and emptied my world of its constant pain, replacing it with relief and hope, I will be there. Not there to watch him die, but afterward, after he is already gone away from this place. This will be a long, long time from now, and, though I am more than twelve years his junior, I will be a very old woman by then. His friends and family, perhaps even his younger wife, will welcome any acquaintances, familiar or unfamiliar, to his funeral. That's what I will be. An acquaintance. The unfamiliar kind.

After the mourners have offered their condolences to one another and after they have, one by one, or clutching one another with bowed heads, made their way to the front of the church to view his aged, unsouled body, then I will go to him, alone, as I had done so many times before. My eyes will be the last to glimpse that beautifully sculptured form before they close his casket and carry him away to lower him into the ground. He will be lying there amidst an artistic array of poignant lines, scars, and wrinkled skin that define every precious moment of his long life. His lips, above and beneath that mossy cover of facial hair, will be drawn up into a small, satisfied smile. His eyes will be closed. His chest will be still and silent. His hands will be folded and set upon his abdomen. He will appear, to me, to be that same alluring antithesis of everything my humdrum existence had been before he entered it, and since. He will look just the way he did when my parched fingers had drunk of him and memorized every inch of his body, soul and spirit. And I will say this to him,

Nothing. I won't say anything at all. I'll just look because I will know he isn't there. I will want to ask him,

Where are you? Why did you go away and leave me alone? But I won't because I will already know that the answer is hidden inside of me. I took him from within his own body all those years ago and preserved him in my most holy of memories. He hasn't been inside his body for a very long time.

shshshshshshshshshsh

The Jains wear face masks to avoid inhaling microscopic insects, and carry a brush to whisk away any living organism that they might otherwise tread or sit upon. Our karmic cycle, they say, depends on acts of violence or non-violence committed in the present lifetime. So if, say, we were unintentionally to squash an ant in one lifetime, we may find ourselves suffering for it in the next lifetime. Did I squash an ant? Is that what I did? I should think that the squashing of an ant would merit being born with a birthmark, not a debilitating illness. But a life is a life is it not? That ant could have been the mayor of Whoville, or the infant son of a peasant ant. They do have a legitimate point, those Jains.

My aunt, my mother's older sister, used to preach that my *illness is a result of sin. Not your sin specifically,* she was careful to point out. *We are just a degenerate race from which nothing good can arise.*

My mother would attempt to defend my infirmity by counter-preaching that I am *a humble and obedient servant who has taken up her cross to follow Jesus.* Either way it's pretty much a lost cause. If I am a descendent of a long line of degenerates, then nothing I do or say or think really matters. One step up, two steps down. Like the game of Snakes and Ladders Wilma and I used to play, descending more than ascending.   She almost always won.

On the other hand, it is a rather romantic notion to think that I have voluntarily chosen to take up my cross to follow the Son of God himself. Up ahead I can barely make him out amid the bellowing crowd, the dust and stones being hurled at him. Someone has gone to the trouble of weaving a crown of thorns and has stuck it into his head. The thorns are in his beautiful eyes too and he is bleeding everywhere from having been flogged and beaten.   I follow a trail of blood, carefully, meticulously, setting my feet in his bloody footprints. It is a long walk to Golgotha, mostly uphill too. Perhaps I should have considered this before I picked up that splintered old cross and started trailing after him. Jesus, way up there ahead of me, stumbling from his own pain and fatigue, sightless from his own blood and wads of mud being heaved at him, is suffering this fate because he has been performing illicit miracles. I, on the other hand, have never performed anything at all, and in fact, am living proof that miracles are a hoax.

The Mormons believe that we choose our path on earth while we are yet in the other realm, Heaven, or some other elusive place. We browse through a catalogue of possible lives, choose one that appears to reap the most benefits for our soul and the souls of those we will meet, then pass through the veil into our mothers' womb, all remembrance of that choice obliterated. I learned this at a funeral. The widow, dressed in cheery daffodil yellows and gold, told me that she took great comfort in knowing that her deceased husband had chosen his course of cancer and early death for a reason and it was not for her to question. They had a four month old baby boy.

Lovely lot, those Mormons. They look after their people and have a worldwide storehouse of goods to be dispersed in times of need. Nice extremists, I'd say.

I guess I am thinking that everybody would like to believe they have the ultimate answer. I don't. I have only questions. Answers would infer absolutes, and I can't say that

I have ever found anything to be perfectly, unequivocally absolute, although there is one thing of which I am quite certain, and that is death. Death is life's one absolute. Unless, of course, you are Enoch or Elijah and then even death is not an absolute. Enoch and Elijah walked with God. In those days, walking with God merited being fetched up to Heaven in a whirlwind or simply disappearance from the earth. I wonder what it is like to walk with God. I would think it something like those terrifying walks by the lake, studying wildflowers with my tutor. Nervous and small you would feel, but important and assured too. You would want to reach out to hold God's hand, but you wouldn't for fear of disapproval or rejection. One couldn't be sure whether or not God did things like that.

I heard that my tutor had died. She'd suffered a massive stroke and was not discovered until the following day. She was found lying in her blue and white rowboat, her body partially immersed in water that had seeped in through minute cracks during the night. The boat had drifted about on the lake for nearly twenty-four hours, then washed ashore near the campground. A boy had found her, a youth of sixteen, fishing off the dock. In the papers it was cited that he'd remarked she was a *sturdy-looking old lady, wrapped in a knitted shawl. She looked so peaceful there, all alone.*

I had never seen my tutor in a knitted shawl. But I suppose everybody must make some changes in their lifetime, great or small.

> *But Lancelot mused a little space*
> *He said, 'she has a lovely face;*
> *God in his mercy lend her grace,*
> *The Lady of Shallot.*

The absorbing heat of the bath has limbered up my

muscles some and eased the ache in my gut, but now I feel weak and faint again. I must be careful standing up. Ever so slowly, and grasping the stainless steel railing my husband installed just for this purpose - just like in old people's bathrooms - I heave myself up to a squatting position first, wait till the blurry waves of dizziness subside to a dull quivering, then raise myself to a standing position, still gripping the railing. When my eyes can focus again, I reach over for the towel and give myself a brisk rub.

I feel refreshed stepping into my clothes. My skin can breathe again after being clogged with itchy oiliness. Apparently, as my doctor says, skin problems are common in people with fatigue disorders. She wrote a prescription for some kind of anti-fungal solution, which I spray onto my face after every cleansing. I've also heard that this sort of skin disorder is a nervous condition, caused by stress, and stress, as everybody knows, is caused by one's inability to handle life's events in a mature, enduring sort of way.

Are you very stressed? is what some doctors used to ask me from behind their guises of white coats and thick medical texts. For awhile I used to reflect offhandedly,

Well, no, not really. I mean, I have nothing to get stressed over. My life is easy and slow, not fast-paced and hectic like so many other people I know.

And this was quite true. I had no time constraints, no boundaries in which to squeeze myself. I did not rise to the rudeness of a buzzing alarm at six a.m. every morning and head out into rush hour traffic. The milieu I followed simply required a leisurely meandering. Later, I said this to those same numb-skulled doctors,

Stressed? Whatever have I got to be stressed over? I LIKE being tired all the time. I LIKE being in pain. I LIKE being nauseated. Feeling sick all the time gives a feeling of pleasure, no, of EUPHORIA! But saying this was exhausting.

My mother's sister has said my fatigue is simply a matter of stress.

And stress is sin, don't you know.

For many, many years, this is what I also believed, not that my physical state was a direct result of personal sin, but that my response to life in general was unhealthy, creating a less than adequate physical condition. I believed I could outdo the fatigue and pain. Yes, I did foolish things like forcing myself to head out into a blizzard to trudge through the snow, thinking this would increase my heart rate, tone up my muscles, increase my appetite, motivate my digestive system, and so on.

I bought a rebounder, on the counsel of my mother, who alleged that Barley Green and regular bouncing on a rebounder were the quintessential tools to a healthy, fit body. I read in the pages of a magazine once that the only equipment a person needed for personal fitness training, aside from proper diet, was a treadmill. So my husband bought a treadmill for me. Then I heard that insomnia was caused by irregular bedtimes, and sleep clinics became all the rage. So I followed those rules for awhile and forced myself to stay awake until midnight, rising every morning at six-thirty after six-and-a-half sleepless hours. Then I read that adults need at least nine hours of solid sleep, so I went to bed at nine o'clock instead and rose after nine-and-a-half sleepless hours.

All these things I have done in an attempt to appease the gods. Once I even conceded to accompanying my aunt to her Tabernacle of Faith meeting. My aunt is in no way condescending, as is one of my in-laws (whose identity in the scheme of my life is relatively unimportant), I must make that clear to myself. She is not insensitive or harsh. But she does have a stupendous and resolute belief in heaven and hell and the two diverging paths that lead to each.

A Sister Something-Or-Other from the Ukraine was in town holding a faith healing meeting. My aunt was adamant that I go along with her, certain I would meet the Lord and be healed. So certain was she that I began to be afraid not to, afraid of her disapproval or rejection of me. Afraid my sins would find me out.

We entered the conference room from the front where anyone at all interested in taking note of the type of patrons who attend these functions could easily do so. Still, in my middle age, which I can now say is upon me, I do not wish to make a spectacle of myself. Yet there I was, knowing that a spectacle I would most assuredly be.

My aunt, smugly thinking that she had broken through some spiritual barrier, or at least, loosened some of the shackles to get me there, had assumed a meek, somewhat accommodating, facade so that I would not be frightened away. She also knew that too much commotion would do me in. My own sense of confusion is one thing, but watching the confusion of others is an overabundance of stimulation that sets me into a self-protective fugue state.

Where would you like to sit? is what she asked as she pulled me through crowds of feet and coats. *Is this all right?* shuffling past a row of knees and overly cheerful faces. I would have preferred to park myself near the back, off-center, so as not to appear overly conspicuous. But since this was my aunt's moment of glory, and after-all, I did aim to please, I followed her through the throngs of immoderately joyful people.

I really feel in my spirit that you're to be healed tonight, said my aunt rather too loudly, I thought, as she removed her jacket, draping it across her knees. *You must believe that Satan will be bound. You will be healed. I sincerely believe that.*

I wanted to believe that. More than anything. There were others there, evidently in need of some sort of healing. A stooped young man in the row in front of us held a cane by his side. His face twitched. One of his hands was withered. It was apparent that he was alone. No one had cajoled him into attending. He must have great faith, I was thinking, with an almost resentful admiration.

There was no pulpit at the front. No stage. But people were beginning to assemble up front with guitars, a banjo, tambourines, an electronic piano, a set of drums. Already my heart had begun to pound in dreaded anticipation of the inevitable joyful noise unto the Lord about to burst forth from those ear-splintering instruments. My aunt, already engrossed in her own inner syncopated rhythm, was beginning to sway and tap her feet on the floor. There were myriad lights, and gushy hugging and excited chattering, when all at once the drummer's first strike resonated throughout the entire building, and the other instrumentalists followed suit. Within moments, the gushiness had metamorphosed into clapping, swaying, bursts of singing and shouting. Those people who were not lame or suddenly jolted into utter terror as I was, stood to their feet. Some even stood on their chairs, waving their arms wildly about, eyes closed, lips moving rapidly. I had never witnessed such a shamozzle of chaos.

My preacher husband had not believed in these charismatic displays of emotion. He had not condoned the gift of speaking in tongues unless there was an interpreter present. *God is a God of order and harmony, not of disorder and confusion,* is what he would often preach. If one of his congregation members wanted healing, he or she would be prayed over by the elders in a dignified, systematic manner. His congregation followed a regimented pattern, preprogrammed and undivergent. We sang traditional hymns with subdued voices, acceptably somber faces, to the accompaniment of organ and sometimes piano. No one dared speak out of turn. In this I agreed with him.

Eventually, the hullabaloo quieted, although it didn't ever cease completely, and a stately looking lady in her fifties emerged from a door behind the drummer. Her shoulder-length hair was dark and radiant. She wore a modest, pastel-blue dress, ankle length, with a white cardigan. A string of some sort of imitation jewels swung rhythmically around her neck and dangled from her ears. Her cheeks were rouged, mouth lip-sticked, yet she displayed an aura of genuineness and believable sincerity.

With raised arms and jubilant voice she welcomed us all,

Greetings in the name of our Lord and Father! Hallelujah! God be praised! A ripple of murmuring, mumbling, singing, swept through the audience. *I bring good news, folks! Good news! Jesus is alive! And He is here today, in this room to bring healing and salvation!*

Again the incoherent mumbo-jumbo, louder this time, undulating in waves around the room. I didn't know whether to laugh or be terribly afraid. Had I dressed appropriately? Would my appearance suggest modesty, worthy of God's healing hand? Perhaps I should button up one more button on my shirt, cross my legs, assume a more demure stance. I should have worn proper shoes, not leather sandals. Someone in my family had once referred to me as a *loose woman*. It'd had something to do with my footwear or lack thereof, though I haven't yet figured out the connection. I would do just about anything to find favor in the eyes of God. I would even wear shoes.

Then the praying began. The lady evangelist called for all those in need of healing to stand. I knew my aunt would not allow me to remain seated. She nudged me, nodded, furrowing her brows in a pleading, assuring sort of gesture. I stood. The evangelist then told us to place our hands on the region of our bodies to be healed. What should I do? Place my hands on my head? Over my heart? A quick scan of inductive reasoning suggested that I place my hands on my stomach, for if God would see fit to repair my faulty plumbing system, other systems should then, logically, begin to function as they should.

She prayed, scanning the audience, without really picking any of us out directly. I forced all of my concentration onto my abdomen, willing thoughts of fear, doubt, and how ludicrous this whole scheme felt to me, aside. I opened every sensory avenue to allow the ignition of heat, or coldness, or tingling, or whatever sense healing was supposed to generate. I closed my eyes, listened, dwelt on every word the evangelist spoke, every breath she breathed. But what if my in-law was right? What if there was a black aura of impenetrable sin shrouding me?

What if devoutly religious people such as this woman had extrasensory perception into the spiritual dimension? What if there were demons perched on my shoulder, as had once been suggested by this same particular in-law? I would need more than a healer. I would need an exorcist and a herd of pigs.

Fear itself, is the only thing to be feared, is what I chided myself.

I leaned on the chair in front of me. I shifted from leg to leg, concentrated on breathing. But to no avail. I had to sit down before the floor wound up in my face. Others were moving forward now, being prayed over with the evangelist's hand on their foreheads. On some was rubbed a dab of oil from a vial in her other hand. A man had gone to the front and was posing behind each of them, his arms outstretched, ready to catch them should the power of God collapse them into masses of jello. Then he would ease them down to the floor, move on to the next, leaving a tidy row of immobile bodies. The calm poise in his stature and the prosaic cast in his expression made it seem as though this was his profession. I'd seen this same matter-of-fact carriage in the Fuller Brush man who had often found himself on our doorstep. He would take a deep breath and on exhalation, sigh,

What'll it be today, Ma'am?

My two years as a conservative preacher's wife had left me with little understanding and rather little scope for appreciation for this sort of melodramatic performance. But had I not come here for healing? Even if Ms. Evangelist up there had to swat the demons off of my shoulders, I would at least give it my best shot. I owed it to my aunt, whose lips were moving, eyelids fluttering, expecting a miracle.

I rose again, but only part way, my knees bent, head lowered, thinking that I might be less of a spectacle if I were shorter, and brushed my way through the rows of knees and feet. Everyone else wore shoes.

Come, Sister, breezed the evangelist's Ukrainian-accented voice. *Come. Come take my hand. No one shall be left out. Eh? Praise the Lord!*

Praise God!

Thank you Jesus!

Is any one of you in trouble? He should pray. Is anyone happy? Let him sing songs of praise. Is any one of you sick? He should call the elders of the church to pray and anoint her with oil in the name of the Lord. And the prayer offered in faith will make the sick person well; the Lord will raise her up. Eh? Praise God?

Praise God! rumbled the echo.

She grasped my hand and began parading me around in circles, round and round we went. She started off like this,

Here is our sister, Jesus, in need of your touch. She is suffering from... poor circulation... and tiredness... and intestinal discomfort...

My hands were frigid as icicles. It didn't take a mortician to figure out I had poor circulation, and it would follow then, that poor circulation would lead to lethargy, and no doubt she had seen me place my own hands on my stomach area to have guessed the intestinal distress. If one proclaimed to be a faith healer and had gathered enough of a reputation, then one would have had to become sensitive and alert to these subtle clues. She prayed and we walked. She did not offer to anoint my brow with oil nor did she place her hand on my forehead. The man behind me was temporarily out of a job.

And then she broke into song again.

He giveth more grace when the burdens grow greater; He sendeth more strength when the labors increase. To added affliction He addeth His mercy; to multiplied trials His multiplied peace.

I wondered why she didn't touch my forehead. Why did she not touch me with the holy oil? What did those other people merit that they should be anointed and I had not? Was it my unbelief? Was there a host of grinning demons perched on my shoulders? Was it that I was hard-hearted, unreceptive, unworthy? Did she think I was feigning like so many others thought of me?

I felt myself blink back a trickle of tears that had leaked, unsolicited, into my eyes. Anyone who had noticed would have decided they were tears of joy, of blessing, relief, not of disappointment. I felt it was my own failure, my own lack of enthusiasm that prevented the good sister here from demonstrating her gift of healing. Faithless people like me did her ministry no good. I was out. Banished. Exiled.

What did I feel? Humiliation? Indignation? Rejection? Sorrow? Loneliness? Vulnerability? I could list a zillion emotions. But maybe I felt nothing. Maybe it was numbness that had finally honed in on an unmoving target.

Looking back now, I begin to see that I have lost all attachment to these events. The connection used to be emotion. But emotions have become a sort of event in themselves, somewhat disconnected from the situation at hand, blunted in a necessary shell of protection. I can, for instance, recall the ride home later that night in my aunt's Buick. She was not her usual chattery self. Maybe she was beginning to succumb to the inevitable skepticism that reigned over the rest of us and was bound to catch her off guard sooner or later. She never said as much, but that was the end of her obstinate speeches about obedience and damnation.

I recall pulling in to Bearberry, her small voice when she asked if I wanted anything and mine saying, *Reese's peanut butter cups please,* and hers saying, *you're mother'll have my hide.* Defeat was in there somewhere, reluctance, and also a weird satisfaction in knowing that I would no longer be her pet project of spiritual reform. Complacency. And maybe an emancipating repose. All of these emotions happened. At some time I must have recorded them into my memory files, but I don't exactly remember ever having these feelings inside of me. They were more like cartoon bubbles above my head.

Now that I think about it, when Wilma and I said good-bye the last time, I don't recall any nameable feelings either. Words that come to mind are: lost, betrayed, abandoned, indebted, yet enveloped in a fuzzy bubble of okayness. There could have been love, devotion, as though I were losing a lover. Maybe I was. Maybe I was in love with Wilma.

My aunt said,

Maybe I am the one who needs healing and vision. Maybe the Lord has opened my eyes. I'm going to find you a doctor who's going to get you well.

shshshshshshshshshshsh

Vision has always been something of an enigma to me. Perhaps my scope is too dim, unfocused, missing critical elements like angle or perspective which provides the portrait with a sense of depth, of wholeness. Or perhaps it is excessively lucid. It is possible to see things too clearly, to know too much. This is true. Ignorance is bliss.

With much wisdom comes much sorrow;
the more knowledge, the more grief.

Some historical theologians claim that the book of Ecclesiastes was scribed by a man named Solomon, king of Jerusalem, who is also purported to be the wisest man in all of history. This wisest of men settled a dispute by offering to slice a child in two in order to appease the two contesting mothers. To me, this seems a reasonable solution. I myself would have done the exact same thing.

This is the problem of knowledge, of foresight, hindsight, insight, and outsight. The book of Ecclesiastes itself is perhaps, the dreariest work ever put down because of its clarity of common sense, of ordinary vision. This is how it begins:

Meaningless! Meaningless!
says the Teacher.
Utterly meaningless!
Everything is meaningless!

137

This is alright with me. But it has been difficult not to project this knowledge onto my children. In time they will consummate their own delusions of meaning. Some people never quite get it. They go through their entire lives seeking consonance, place, belonging, thinking it is there to be found, as though meaning has been something misplaced a long time ago, in some other era before language had begun to erode it into an invaluable commodity, like gold, or the idea of gold. There have been scads of books written on the subject. How to Find Personal Meaning. Existentialism and Meaning. The Meaningful Experience. The Unheard Cry for Meaning. And so on. I find all these attempts at reducing the agony far too private a matter for public consumption.

It is nauseatingly difficult, for instance, when you consider that the sun takes approximately two-hundred-and-forty-million earth years to complete one orbital cycle in its path around this particular galaxy, to impose anything of significance onto this dust particle we call the earth. Earth. Even the word becomes hollow when you say it. Earth. Erth. Irth. Urth. Rth.

And yet, I have taken some kind of captious amusement from watching the humanoid species of this earth conduct themselves. I have, at this point, pretty much given up this practice, but not long ago I would still watch them, like looking through the wrong end of a telescope, far away, myself extracted from the scene.

Down at the store sometimes I would watch them through this abstracted spectrum. They would be buying butter, matches and fishhooks, or others would be pumping gas and antifreeze into salt-glazed vehicles whose dazed passengers asked for restroom keys, and spoke to one another with strained effort.

Pop?
Coke.
Money?
Pocket.

Which one?
Front, left.
Paper?
None left.

There were those who paid for the gas and those who collected the money. There were those who came in later in the day and swept, mopped up muddy footprints, restocked dusty shelves with more dusty products. There were also those who just stood around in huge green gumboots, posing with Styrofoam coffee cups and smoldering cigarettes. These ones interested me the most, the stationary figures, the ones with nowhere to go, nowhere to be. I felt they were closer to the truth than the ones always on the move, buying, selling, peeing. These ones were probably closer to realizing that their lives meant dick-squat.

Yet I hold an esteemed admiration for all of these beings. Obviously they still care about something. I am envious of all these people. The people who care. I can't remember what it's like to care about anything.

I suppose I shouldn't judge though. I should imagine that without pain, or with less pain even, there might be something to care about. I fear I have become indelibly selfish with my pain.

And so I would pack up my mental telescope and go home to ponder.

Lately I have been able to see myself. Not as one looks in the mirror, mindless of one's own existent appearance. But as other people might see me. From a distance, not from behind the subjectivity of these eyes. I am beginning to understand the vacancy people read into my stature or my inexpressiveness sometimes. They see that I have a finely contoured jaw bone, when I had always thought my face roundish, indistinct. They see that my cheekbones are high on my face, but with a hint of elegance and form, not gaunt or protuberant as I had supposed. I have always thought my chin round, almost babyish, but now I see that it is not. Rather, it seems to meld into the jaw line, which reaches with fine upward strokes to my hairline. I have also thought of my hair as thin, flat, bothersome and dull, except for the warmth it provides. But now, from this distant stance, I see that my hair is multi-colored, light on top, reddish brown streaking through it and a blonde patch in my bangs. It appears to be alive, like Medusa's head of serpents. At thirty-five the skin of my neck has the tendency to pull beyond its elasticity, creating a sort of sinewy refinement. You would want to see this neck emerging from a dark velour, V-necked sweater to capture its complete essence of femininity. My shoulders are delicate, yet not fragile. I look like a woman. This is what I find most puzzling. I do not feel like a woman. I have never been tall enough to allow myself the benefits of having the whole woman status. I've always shopped in the girls' section, or boys', at thrift stores. I've always worn scruffy clothing; frayed jeans, skirts that hang on me like curtains, men's flannel shirts and long, bulgy underwear, baggy, holy socks, or no socks. There has never been anything woman about me, not that I could see.

I now see the abandoned, purposeless obscurity in my sea-gray eyes; the way I stand, inerect, Raggedy-Ann shoulders drooping forward and down slightly, the way my floppy legs jut out beneath me preventing my bottom from scraping along the ground; my knobby knees, like burls, or benign disfigurements; creaky, stiff joints; imprecise movements; my head inclined to one side as if immortalized in a perpetual plight of puzzlement.

I guess it's no wonder they wonder about me.

I see myself at about ten years of age, in the middle of a swinging bridge above the James River. I am wearing my orange and purple bell-bottoms and a hooded sweatshirt. My father is below, calling out fatherly caution. I am somewhere below, not quite on the ground, but above the rushing river. I am not anywhere on that bridge. But I see myself, nevertheless. I see the pale threads of my hair swinging out in all directions so there must be parts of me on all sides. I see that I am leaning precariously over the lax rope, looking down over the gushing, tumbling water. With envy? I can sense my father's concern. From behind it looks as though I am about to topple over the edge. A front view suggests that I am reaching for the water, which is at least twenty feet below. Why would I be reaching for the water?

I spend too much time in front of the mirror these days. What I see there fascinates me on account of a recent, acute awareness of detail. Again, this seems to be an excess of both intrinsic and extraneous vision. The images don't vanish when I close my eyes. They expound, dazzling me with fastidious intricacies. This worries me some. Am I becoming schizophrenic, for instance, lost in a wilderness of irrelevant detail and spasms of modulating thoughts? Are my silences delineations of catatonic seizures?

I have considered the possibility of hypersensitivity. The inability to screen out unimportant sensations. I am totally aware, for instance, of every single breath I take. But why shouldn't I be? Breath is our very existence.

I can also feel, with explicit clarity, the sensation of space against my skin. The minute hairs on my skin vibrate with every move I make. It is not unlike swimming, except heavier, more cumbersome, without the comfort of the water's closeness to keep you from falling. I have never been fond of wind because the sensation is far too stimulating and seems to upset the delicate balance of the space in which I move and breath. It steals my breath.

I am aware of the sensation of swallowing, how food is propelled down my throat in waves of peristaltic action, so slowly it seems stuck and I would choke if I did not avert my awareness away. I can feel my stomach bounce and sag with food, like a trampoline with too many bodies on it. My intestines, a great sluggish earthworm, move slowly, tense, spasm, move forward, backward, halt, harden, and so on.

I am aware of the ovulation process. I know exactly where the egg lies, the precise moment when it breaks away from the ovary and propels itself through the fallopian tube, seeking a companion, seeking a home. My insides feel red, inflamed, hot. My body contorts, languidly abiding the torture of its femaleness. There is nowhere for the egg to go now, so it just disintegrates, becomes part of the interstitial parade through my body. I can feel this, the disintegrating. It is a pop, sharp, jagged, then dull, spreading outward into my pelvis.

I am aware of the constant pounding of my heart, the pulsing in every vein and artery. The main artery between the parting of my ribcage protrudes, pulsating in hyper-dynamic rhythms. If I lie on my back I can watch it thrump around. I like to imagine there is an infant alien in there, incubating, feeding off the energy of my body, squirming in preparation for its birth which will be my death.

I am even aware of the microscopic parasites that wriggle around in the fluid on my eyeballs. Often I watch them, their black heads and the transparent outlines of their bodies and tails. I hope I am a good home to them.

I would like to be silent again, if I could, for this constant bombardment of thought is alienating me from the external world in which my corporeal form still exists. It astounds me, this protracted, enigmatic existence which I seem to grip with a baffling, stoic acceptance. But my silences have become turbulent. There seems to be very little space left in the web of convoluting passageways that constitutes my metaphysical being. Even my dreams are not exempt. My husband dreams of animals, of tracking moose on bicycles down stumpy cut lines, and of wrestling giant rainbow trout in his underwear. But my dreams are perforated with stench, clutter and cacophony, induced by constant nausea, bowel spasms and a rank taste in my mouth. I dream of drowning in a lake of Pepto Bismol, or swallowing writhing snakes, or impaling myself on my own petrified intestines. Or falling because I never learned to fly. I whispered this to my doctor once, ashamed of what I perceived as a weakness. She said,

142

People who are tortured have nightmares.

There is a dream catcher above my bed, barren, uninhabited like a deserted spider's web.

These thoughts of mine generally flash before me in a series of vivid images, no longer defined by the superfluity of words or sentences. Even my pain has become just another dimension of my existence so that it cannot be conceived in tangible rhetoric.

I must quicken my pace now. The kids will be home in only an hour and what have I done? There is laundry to do, floors to be swept, mopped. I should dust the piano, wipe down the television, the table, straighten the blankets on my bed. I strive to establish a semblance of order of my own to minimize the disorder of children and husband. My evenings are spent in my bedroom, reading, wedged in by pillows and blankets, my heating pad packed into the small of my back. I have a noisemaker, which sounds like a fan, blocking out other distracting sounds. I have a bottle of water on the bedside table; a lamp; a stack of books; paper and pencil in case I should want to draw a picture, which I never have, but the very possibility of an impromptu inspiration intrigues me; sleeping medication which I rarely take; Gravol, of which I take a lot; tubes of Mentholatum chap stick and hydrocortisone cream; an array of candles, most of them burnt down to blobs of wax; a matchbook; and gobs of clingy dust. This is what my life has been reduced to.

I suppose this reduction has come about by the annihilation of choices. There was a time, not too many years ago, when I found it easier to overlook the pain. Perhaps overlook is the wrong word. It was a sort of penitence I would induce upon myself. There were so many babies happening and so many other family members with such a multitude of things to be done and not enough pairs of hands. My greatest ambition was to give of my time and meager resources, thinking that this ambition would be appreciated, if not reciprocated. Again, this assumption of mine was clearly unfounded, downright stupid of me. One of my greatest delights, at the beginning, was just to hold my nieces and nephews, snuggling their softness against my cheeks. The smell of their babyness and the blurry innocence in their eyes made me feel as though I could recover some of the bond I'd misplaced with my own firstborn son. But that one small indulgence of mine was ripped away from me with more brutal force than if I'd been smacked in the face with a two-by-four.

You don't touch my child! You're not his mother! I know when my own child needs to be held and by whom, and I'd appreciate it if you'd stop interfering. My job as a mother is to protect the welfare of my children and that means keeping you away from them. I can't keep you away from our other nieces and nephews, but I surely have say over what occurs in my own family! I won't have a crazy woman doting over my children!

I think I must have been projecting my own desperate need for help onto others' intentions. I was doing unto others as I would have done unto myself. If only someone would take the time to assist me in these days of often unbearable pain. But would I accept it? No, likely not. I would smile and say,

No, that's all right. I'm fine. Of course, no one, as yet, has ever offered, aside from my mother. I think I would be dumbstruck.

I bear no resentment. Why should I? What possible benefit could resentment have on the delicate fabric of our family relations? Did not the people of ancient Rome gather in huge coliseums to watch with glee the gladiators bludgeon one another to death? Or were not prisoners tossed into an arena of hungry lions? The crowds went wild over the humans that resisted the most, the ones who screamed and fought, terrorized to death. The ones that resigned themselves to their fate, allowing their limbs to be torn apart without a struggle, there was no glory in this. People love a good fight. Is this even a fair comparison? What have I got to gripe about, really?

Although I do not share them, I suppose I can understand where her invective sentiments might be coming from. There are a million other Canadians out there, besides myself, who are not only misunderstood, but are also stigmatized and penalized for having Chronic Fatigue Syndrome or other related troubles. The thing is, those of us who live with this indisposition are too exhausted to speak out. We are repudiated as displaying hypochondriac behavior. Most of us have been coerced, through a combination of physical disabilities and social rejection, into a state of enforced reclusion. We bear a heavy banner of social aloofness, which appears to others as self-centeredness. But most of us are too tired to defend ourselves.

We have no need of defense.

My choices have been dramatically altered as a result of this stigma. But it is an infamy I will bear with dignity, however private and concealed that may be. At our family get-togethers, I watch her with curious admiration, the exaggerated silences she ostentatiously displays in my presence, the exactness of dominion she exhibits over her children who eye me with inquisitive apprehension.

My mom doesn't like you for real! is what the ingenuous four-year-old tells me with a proud gleam.

And I reply, with a secretive ruffle of my fingers through his fine hair, *I know. And that's okay. You know why?*

Why?

Because I love you. And I love your mother, too, that's why.

You do?

Uh, huh

I'm gonna tell her that.

I haven't yet spoken with anyone else afflicted with this

drastic limitation of choices, the browbeating scorn, rejection, humiliation, etc. The diagnosis I received only four years ago came about by a series of exclusions.

It's not this and it's not that, and it's probably not this either, and so on. The kindly psychologist, in his report, wrote that *a diagnosis of Chronic Fatigue syndrome would seem warranted.* The internal specialist gave me an eighteen-second exam of the fibromyalgia tenderpoints, then hurriedly handed me a half-page blurry photo copy of Chronic Fatigue Syndrome symptoms on his way out the door to a golf tournament. There was a phone number on the page. I called it. A recording of a woman's voice trickled weakly through the line. It sighed,

I'm sorry, but most of us are too tired to answer your calls today. Please leave us your name and phone number and a detailed message and someone will return your call. Remember - you are not alone.

It was three months before that call was returned, but in the meantime, I felt hopeful for the first time. Although it was only a recording, I felt akin to that voice, touched by its sincerity, its pain, honesty. It didn't matter that she didn't know who I was. She had told me that I wasn't alone. Even my aloneness wouldn't seem so solitary anymore. I almost felt worthy of my pain. Although now that I am actually thinking this, it seems absurd, funny almost. Why should we think that without suffering our lives would be incomplete? If this were true, then I should be about as complete as one can get. I suppose this is just another illusion of hope. But as I said, I believe in illusions.

Yet it was two more years before my name finally migrated to the top of a list of fifteen hundred.

She is kind and sympathetic, my doctor. She tells me that I am allergic to ninety percent of the foods that I eat. But what am I to do about it? She tells me that I have a contracted blood volume, as little as half the normal blood volume for a healthy adult my size. (Sometimes I like to think that I am a closeted vampire.) To increase the blood volume I must eat the foods I cannot eat (Or suck blood from some unsuspecting victim). The diagnostic summary for my case goes like this, in condensed form:

Chronic Fatigue Syndrome

Fibromyalgia

Neurally Mediated Hypotension

Documented Episodic Hypotension with multiple systolics in the 70s

Irritable Bowel Syndrome

Leaky Gut

Protein Energy Malnutrition secondary to poor tolerance to food due to chronic illness

Abnormality of the right Iliac Artery with an extremely large and palpable artery on the right and a diminished pulse on the left

Possible Narcolepsy

Post-Prandial Hypotension and Tachycardia leading to severe fatigue after meals, and so on.

But what am I to do?

She also tells me that the prognosis for recovery is slim in lifelong cases such as mine, although not entirely unattainable.

What we aim for, in your case, is to ease the discomfort, which we will do. But you must be patient. You have shown an exceptional degree of understanding, motivation and persistence in dealing with these issues.

She is a gracious lady, soft brown eyes, an unhurried demeanor, clearly gifted in the art of listening. Something about her reminds me of Wilma, which sets me instantly at ease in her presence. I believe her.

The kids have just banged their way through the door, coats and shoes and school bags flying every which way. I take another deep breath, the fullness of which cascades down my windpipe, inflating my lungs. I imagine that I am a breath

147

being drawn into a cavernous expanse, leaving no space untouched. If I were a breath of air, I would caress, transform, heal everything I could feel with my vaporous fingers.

Hi Mom! What's for supper?

Food. Lately, I speak in monosyllables, protecting every particle, every atom of evanescent breath. But my daughter has just reached her full potential of concrete operational thought. Nothing is abstract.

What kind of food?

Slop.

What kind of slop?

Good slop.

MOM!

Okay, roast and potatoes and carrots. The usual slop.

Yum, can we eat?

Soon as your father gets home.

Aaww.

The TV flicks on. The fridge gets opened, and shut, then opened again. There is a flurry of rustling activity behind the open fridge door, gulps, chomps, spills, *whoops,* the door gets slammed hurriedly. Cupboards open, then slam, TV channels get flipped through, bedroom doors flung open, banging against the wall, a stream of squawky voices,

Where'd'ya put my Discman?

Didn't put it nowhere!

Did too! You were in my room again!

Prove it!

Get out!

You get out!

You get out! It's your turn to get the eggs anyway.

MOM!

I switch my noisemaker onto the high setting, slither down into my blankets. How many more years of this? Six, at least? I must not let myself think this way. It's not their fault. Children should be allowed to be children. It isn't right that I

148

should hide away in my bedroom like this. How would I have felt, as a child, if my mother had retreated to the semi-privacy of her bedroom every time I walked into the room? What if she had lived her life behind a closed door the way I do, shutting the world from her own self-administered psychosis? It isn't right.

I struggle to my feet again. What did I eat today? Just some nuts, I think. They were in my coat pocket. I remember munching on them earlier, before my nap, as I recall, tossing a few over the fence for the chickens as I rumbled past on the quad. My insides should be fairly unobstructed then. I should be able to make it through supper, dishes. Maybe I should have some yogurt, or a banana. No, bananas cramp me up. No bananas. Yogurt with some orange juice concentrate, just a little, enough to add flavor, not enough to create a haven of acidity down there in my gut.

I go to the fridge, open it. Raspberry jam has been glopped on the shelf. I sigh, restrain my annoyance, trudge to the sink, wet a cloth, trudge back, wipe it up, throw the cloth across the room where it plops somewhere near the sink. A pail of yogurt is hauled from the top shelf. I made it just yesterday. I do these things, make pails of yogurt and other concoctions, drearily, without thinking. I don't know why. Yogurt, bread, muffins, chocolate chip cookies, pots of chili, stew, ice cream sometimes with crumbled Oreo cookies, etc. I even got the recipe for woopy pies from Wilma's white-haired mother. These things have become my penitence now. What else would be acceptable? This is the compensation my children and husband receive in exchange for a mother or wife.

A bowl is retrieved from the dish-drainer. A spoonful of yogurt is blobbed into it, and a teaspoon of orange concentrate. I lick the spoon. Such luxury. Smooth, icy, tartly sweet. While this mixture is spooned slowly, methodically into my mouth, running thickly down my throat, cooling my insides, three plates are pulled from the cupboard, spoons and forks from the drawer, which I see is in need of reorganizing. Tomorrow. The roast is forked out of the slow cooker, plunked onto a cutting board, sliced into thick chunks. Potatoes and carrots and onions are heaped into an empty ice cream bucket. The juice from the roast is poured into a saucepan, into which is also dumped a flour and water paste, some salt, pepper, dash of garlic powder, basil, dash of cayenne, and then whisked into a lumpy gravy.

First it settles into my lower back, then creeps upwards, through my spine and around my inner organs, clenching them with an unrelenting grip. I grasp the edge of the counter, feet apart, pull myself forward and downward, stretch out the soreness. It. Like my pain is a Thing now. An entity of its own, slithering about inside my body, ensuring no part of me is left untouched by its engulfing, tormenting claws. Spidering down into my legs, pressing into my knees, my ankles. It feels as though my face has fallen off, into the gravy. My ears hurt. My toenails hurt.

The TV is blaring. I should refrain from asking the kids to turn it down, but they will understand. After-all, it is a small sacrifice. They can do this for me if I can feed them.

Kids? Could you turn it down just a tad?

Mom, it's as low as it gets without turning it to mute.

There I go again. Misjudging. Sounds, lights, movements. All these things are magnified to ten times. I see that the lights are all off in the house. I can't very well tell them to turn down the lights. Again, I have lost all sense of objectivity.

There are no structured meal times around here. Not anymore. Years ago, while I still had a whiff of strength, or was more tolerant, we used to eat together. We had a tablecloth, pale blue with crocheted edges. We had place mats, woven, multicolored lines, frayed edges. I used to set the table, plates, glasses, forks, knives, spoons, salad bowls, cloth napkins sometimes. I used to set the food out in separate bowls, with serving spoons. We used to pray before each meal, holding hands. We used to do these sorts of family things. Now, quite often meals don't make it from pot to plate. They

150

feed themselves straight from the skillet sometimes, on the counter, stove, couch, community tea towel to wipe their grimy hands. As long as they have an unobstructed view of the television. The Simpsons is on at five o'clock every day. Sometimes I lie on the couch and watch it with the kids. It amuses me, the only thing left that amuses me. This is sad.

I'm sorry. I'm sorry. Have I said this out loud? If so, not loud enough to be heard. But I am sorry. I shouldn't be here. I am not into palmistry, but if you were to look at the lifeline on both of my hands, you would notice that it is shadowed by a transparent, wispy line that runs parallel. This offshoot tributary occurs early in its life and persists, uncrossed, to the base of my thumb where it ends abruptly while the main line squirrels right around my thumb and onto the back of my hand. I shouldn't say it ends. It just isn't there anymore, not that I can see. If I could follow this trajectory backwards through time, back to where it branches away from the main line, I might be able to pinpoint the exact moment it crossed over. Was it a choice, something I could have resisted or embraced? Was it folly on my part? Did I neglect to pull a toque over my head one day during that warm, wet spring of 1975? Did I breathe in someone's contaminated air space? It could have been living on the end of a pen that someone else had used and I picked up, chewed on. It could have been a cat. I suppose it might even have been the unflushed toilet at Wilma's house. Probably it was none of these things at all.

How I long for solitude now. I no longer search for pleasure of any kind, really. Just quietness. Not complete noiselessness. The nighttime sounds of the prairies kind of quietness. Sounds that should be there. Not television, voices of bickering children, even the sound of a doting husband is overstimulation these days.

Are you all right, Pica? Are you tired? What kinds of moronic questions are those?

Pica: Close relatives of rabbits. Common near

rockslides at high elevations in the mountain region, living in isolation from one another. Active throughout the year, it spends the majority of the warmer months gathering food for winter. Picas have the unusual habit of drying harvested vegetation in the sun (like hay) before storing it.

My husband often calls me this. *Pica, My Pica.*

I hear his truck pull into the driveway. Door slams. Door opens and shuts. Thumping of boots being placed against the wall. Coveralls being shed and hung on a wall hook.

Can we eat now, Dad?
Where's Mom?
In her bedroom.
Did she make anything?
Yup. Roast and potatoes.
And carrots and gravy.
Turn the TV off first.
Aaww.

I can hear them, above the constant hum of my noisemaker. My family. Mine. The one I created without meaning to, without knowing. The man I love, or once loved, or would love if I had the strength. The children I bore, not thinking what a dreary world it was to bring them into. It isn't fair. They deserve more. They deserve something. I can't think about love right now. The word love itself is draining. It connotes commitment, affection, response, purpose, all of which suggest activity of both mental and physical properties.

The bedroom door opens a crack. I set my eyes upon the lanky silhouette of my angel as he watches me. His eyes have not adjusted to the darkness of our bedroom. He doesn't know my eyes are open and I am looking at him wishing there were something to say to ease his sympathy for me. He thinks I am asleep. This is a practical notion and my husband is a practical man. After-all, most people, lying alone in the darkness of their own bedroom, swathed in a heap of blankets, would be asleep. What other purpose would there be? Who would just lie there, doing nothing, while there is so much to be done and seen and spoken and heard and tasted and felt?

I begin to rock, as I sometimes do. It gives my body something else to do, other than throb with pain. Pain, my constant companion. It does not abuse me. It does just what it is supposed to do. Have I begun to love my pain, to surrender to it? It is not unlike a childhood imaginary friend, although it is not imaginary and it has many names. I speak to it, bearing no ambivalence. I will it away. But my will is weak, ineffectual. Sometimes it is the mental agony of injustice that hurts more than the actual physical pain. Why couldn't it have been something simple, like AIDS or cancer? Certain. Believable. Something with a convincing beginning, tangible choices for treatment, and a marked ending, something to anticipate, rather than this remote, vague sway of limbo.

I could go take another bath, but my skin becomes so itchy with dryness I sometimes lie awake all night filing my fingernails on dry skin. Also, I try to conserve. My husband doesn't go to work every day just to pay the heating bill so I can soak in the bathtub all day.

You would think there would be a dent on my side of the bed. My body feels so heavy sometimes, chained to the mattress. I'm not sure where it is, my body. I see an arm, a leg, a foot, but they don't appear to be attached to my body because my limbs are made of stone while these ones are standard appendages, not mammoth as they feel. I watch my diaphragm rise and fall wondering how and why it keeps on moving like that, almost effortlessly it appears, when it feels as though someone has piled sandbags on top of me.

I used to want it to stop. I believed my doctor when she said,

Two years, just give me two years and I'll have you taking that cross-country bicycle trip you've been talking about.

When was that? About two years ago? I don't think about getting better anymore. I don't think about an ending to

153

the pain. It is too much trouble to want things, too wearying. I'll just lie here. Tomorrow will be better.

I watch the clock, red, electronic numbers, changing one minute at a time, one line at a time. It frustrates me, this clock. It stares at me, jeers at me, minute after minute, hour after sleepless hour, reminds me that more than twenty years have tick-tocked away in this fashion. Time flits about in odd contortions. A single day will seem endless, like today, and yet a whole year will rush past with astonishing alacrity. I melted a clock once, the one with the mini stellar sphere. Every night I would place it face down on top of my lamp to light it up. But one night I left it too long. The plastic sphere melted, twisted into a contorted ribbon shape, and would no longer rotate. It still kept time, but its true value had been depleted. Eventually I exchanged it for a regular clock radio.

shshshshshshshshshshsh

Value. What is value but attachment?

I can't seem to find the value in my being a mother or a wife, or an anybody, for that matter. My children apologize to me. They say things like, *Sorry for being so noisy, Mom.* Or, *Sorry the house is so messy, Mom. We'll clean it up.* Or, *Sorry for bothering you.*

Those apologies are acceptable. Normal, to an admissible extent. But when they become self-debasing, like this, *Sorry you have to put up with us.* Or, *Sorry we were born, Mom,* then I know I have gone too far. But what am I to do? Even my husband apologizes for things that are not within his range of influence.

Oh, Honey, I'm so sorry you don't feel well.

Or my aging mother, *Oh why didn't I see it all those years ago? I'm so sorry, Honey. It hurts me to see you so tired. I feel so helpless. So helpless. A mother shouldn't be helpless.*

But I don't want any of them to be sorry. I am the one to be apologetic. I shouldn't be here. It is unjust, my gloomy complexion dictating, stifling their every move the way it does. My husband promises me better times.

Next year you'll have a basement. I'll build you a soundproof room. All yours, with lots of soft lights and pillows and a TV and a library.

But what good would that do? My children need a mother, not a ghost who lives under the floor.

Their suffering has been no less or greater than mine. This I know. I read, somewhere, an analogy of the magnitude of suffering. It went like this:

> *If a certain quantity of gas is pumped into an empty chamber, it will fill the chamber completely and evenly, no matter how big the chamber. Thus, suffering completely fills the human soul and conscious mind, no matter whether the suffering is great or little. Therefore, the size of human suffering is absolutely relative.*

It isn't fair. It really, really isn't fair.

So I have thought it through, many, many times. Yes, I, too, am methodical in my contemplations. I have thought, in conscientious detail, of every conceivable method and the many trajectories of its aftermath. I could follow Peggy and her choice of pills upon pills. But Peggy, even though she was ill, probably had a more substantive digestive system than I. Pills just wouldn't work for me. And it would be a horrible mess to have to clean up. I would throw up and throw up and throw up some more. By then I would have been discovered and taken to the hospital where my stomach would no doubt be pumped and I would throw up some more. The visualization of this scene is not at all appealing.

Violence has never been my strong point. I wouldn't even know how to load a firearm even though my husband has endeavored to teach me on many occasions. Besides, there is always the possibility of missing. I know of a fellow over in Olds. He lives in a home for severely handicapped people. I have seen him behind the panes of his living room window, which is also his bedroom and dining room window. His face is mangled, looks somewhat like pizza with black olives, and there he sits in his wheelchair. I have also seen him riding the

Handibus to and from the mini-mall. Rumor has it that he'd had rather poor aim and ended up blasting off half his face and severing all motor nerves. Now he is a quadriplegic. No thanks.

Blood has a certain mystical, romantic flavor to it though. Surely bleeding to death couldn't hurt much, just the initial sting and shock, then the slowly falling asleep. I should think it rather warm and dreamy. I could pour a hot bath. I could do it in the bathtub, surrounded by bubbles. I can imagine how the water would look after my blood has begun to ooze out of me, swirling in lovely pinkish rivulets in the soft mounds of bubbles. But I suppose there is a certain sense of violence attached to slicing oneself too, unless it could be done accidentally. Unfortunately, I rarely have accidents anymore and certainly none quite so injurious. Over all of these clumsy years, I have learned to watch my step with meticulous precision. I only bump into walls and stumble over my own feet.

During the winter, when blankets of snow cover the earth, I have often imagined myself an aged Native woman heading out into the night, knowing my time has come. It is time to offer myself back to the earth. The land of the living has no more need of my skills, my wisdom. My seed has dried. I am ready to be planted. Or like an animal, wandering off where it can die peacefully alone. I am afraid that this too, would meet its challenges. My body is far too skilled in hypothermic action. It knows how and when to go into hibernation. I could lay out there in -40C for a week and finally give up and go home. But I wouldn't know. I have never tried this.

Perhaps the only option left to me is carbon monoxide. The garage is small, just enough for my blazer and me. I could get the kids off to school, run out and start it up, close the garage doors, lie down somewhere and hopefully, eventually be overcome by toxic fumes. I wouldn't do it exactly this way. Of course I would have to get an early start, in case my body also rejected toxicity. I would first check the gas gage. I wouldn't want the engine to go sputtering and quitting on me.

I would take with me, some water, and like Peggy, some Gravol. I wouldn't want to become too nauseated in the process. I would close the garage door, but open all the blazer doors. Perhaps I would lie the back seat down, bring pillows, blankets. I may as well be comfortable. I would bring a book. Why would I bring a book? What could I possibly want to read? And what would be the point in reading it? I suppose that it wouldn't be much different from the way I lie here and read day after day, propped up on pillows, with my heating pad on maximum, feeling nauseated and sleepy. No, it wouldn't be any different, except that I would know that I was on my way this time. I wouldn't know for sure, though. I could only hope. I would cross my fingers.

What will it be like, dying, being dead? I suppose it won't be like anything. Sometimes I have actually gone to sleep. Medicated, of course, but the point is, I have been asleep. There is nothing in that sleep. I look at the clock when I wake and realize that four, maybe five hours have passed in that nothing state. It must be like this, except you don't wake up and realize that time has gone by. You just won't wake up. This doesn't sound too bad. It is not appealing, really, because there is always a certain relief, a certain assurance when you do wake to look at the clock. I expect that many of those in labor camps during war times felt much the same way. Perhaps they didn't want to wake. But in waking, they could at least know they had.

I allow myself to think this way sometimes. I have to. These contemplations are my only glimpses of hope, of respite, something tangible in an obscure landscape of perpetual ambiguity. Sureness. They are gifts to myself. They are tidy, these thoughts, whole and complete, yet small enough to contain. They are graceful and tuned like the fine, synergistic movements of ballet as seen from a distance. Up close, of course, you might detect the imbalance; the tremoring muscles, beads of perspiration, protruding veins and sinewy, taut ligaments. But from a credible distance, what you get is flawless balance, ease, composure. These thoughts dance through my mind in much the same way, with prudent enthusiasm, pacific curiosity. They don't whirl about like so many of my other meanderings. These thoughts have form, substance, direction.

No, it wouldn't do, carbon monoxide. It wouldn't be right, them having to find me like that, haul me out of the blazer, turn off the motor, re-open all the doors. How would he carry me inside? Would he cradle me like a child? Would he place one of his strong arms beneath my knees, the other cradling my head and carry me into the house, lay me on the couch? Would he brush my hair, wash my face, caress my cold hands? Would he kiss me? What would it sound like, in the house? Probably there would be quiet, the kind of quiet I have longed for.

Who would make supper? Would anyone remember to feed the chickens?

No, that wouldn't do at all. I shall be like Enoch. I shall just disappear. Perhaps a combination of methods would accomplish the task. Yes, tomorrow, after I have seen the kids off to the school bus, I will take a walk. The walk I would have taken today had I not lain down instead. I will go to the river. In my pocket I will carry a bottle of water, some Gravol tablets, and my sleeping pills which so far, haven't made me sick. I will wear my snowsuit, even though the temperature could be in the teens tomorrow. I wouldn't want to feel cold right away and have to come back to lie on my heating pad. I will walk down the gravel road, cross the highway, cut across the field, climb through fences the way Wilma and I did the day I broke my arm. Probably I will rip my snowsuit on the barbed wire, but it won't matter.

I will think of Wilma while I walk. I will think of living inside her body behind that beautiful face, those freckles. I will imagine the world through those brown button eyes.

I will keep walking. I will approach the tree line and enter the forest. I will imagine what it is like to be a leaf, touched by frost, shedding its deep green, transforming into a kaleidoscope of soothing hues, loosening its grip on the branch, drifting towards the earth, settling among a family of leaves already established there on the ground, among twigs, insects, falling asleep.

I will keep walking. Soon I will reach the edge of the precipice leading down to the river. I will grasp branches, roots, swing myself down. I will feel like Tarzan, or Jane. I will hear only the river bubbling its way towards another river, and another, then out to sea. I shall hum the song I once learned in Sunday School,

Come to the river, there is a vast supply; come to the river that never shall run dry.

Shall I play awhile? Shall I press my face through the surface of that cold water and blow bubbles? Should I play skip rock? Should I take a dry branch and poke it around in the mud, the sand? Write something? What would I write? My name? The date? Draw a happy face?

I will become a poet in my last minutes. I shall write poems in my mind, maybe in the sand. Something like this,

There's dancer in my head
her hands tug at the stars
her eyes follow the moving chasms of time
never missing a single beating moment
her feet like butterflies' wings
in rhythms of immaculate intonations
and never quite touch the earth of my mind
yet her footprints are there
carved into the sand's surface
without chisel or knife
in perfect unpremeditated choreography
wistful is her breath
and her song is silent and clear

There's a dancer in my head

160

and when the dancer ceases to dance
I shall cease to be

Of course I should not romanticize this any more than is necessary. Really, it is all just a process. Just another process, one that requires energy. But the energy requirement will be a one way affair this time. I won't have to calculate the return energy. So many things I haven't even begun because of this two-way stream. I quit driving in to town because there was always coming back with a load of groceries I had to worry about. Holidays were never very festive in our household because what went up had to come down; Christmas wreaths and trees and the bother of sweeping up the shedded pine or spruce needles, or Christmas presents wrapped in plastic Co-op bags to avoid the bother of a sea of wrapping paper shreds and tape stuck to everything; Halloween and messy, unscrubbable paints or carved pumpkins and the bother of kids whining about keeping the mushy, rotted things all year; Easter egg hunts and the bother of stepping on overlooked eggs or listening to the arguing about whose basket is smaller; Canada Day and the bother of expensive, deafening firecrackers or going to town for a midnight wiener roast and more ear-splitting firecrackers and noisy children.

I think, if I were a child, I would want to do all these things. I would want a mother who would do these things with me.

So long have I been twisting myself up with remote possibilities based on someone else's potential. All these years of arduous assembling. Did I think I was Hercules, beyond ruin, tireless, indefatigable? But now the disassembling process will begin. I will start by unfurling myself from that tight wad of desire. I will let them all escape - all those women I so desperately wanted to be. All the lives I wanted to live. I will watch them go, one by one, grasping hands, dancing, singing, playing. They are all very beautiful. Polished and long-suffering like my tutor; nurturing and willful like my

161

mother; fiery, potent like my special in-law; proud and sensible like my confidante, Peggy; gracious, simple like Wilma's mother; agile, easy, silly and compassionate like Wilma. All of them have parts of Wilma. They could all be Wilma, all of her many irresistible components enmeshed into one.

These I will liberate and it will okay to let them go. What right had I to inhibit them, to hold them captive with my fierce lust? What might I have been, were it not for this stray wisp of a body? Would I have been capable of realizing my potential? Or are my cravings only a derivative of ill health? Might I have gone about my daily business with the same humdrum mindlessness the rest of the world displays? Would I have gone to the store to buy butter and matches and fishhooks, would I have pumped gas and antifreeze into my blazer, would I have swept up the residue of those who bought and sold and pumped? Would I have joined the baby-sitting pool and gone to the Christmas bazaars and faithfully sent out birthday cards? Would certain family members have been more agreeable, accepting? Might they have liked me a little?

My husband often says this,
If only you had your health...
I say nothing in return, but inside I scowl, though not at him, rather, at the idea. What good does it do us to say, or even think, *if only you had your health...* as though our whole existence depends upon my health. I suppose, in a way, it does. In a very big way. Like now, I assume. How do my children cope with their experience of having a mother? This experience is so ingrained into their childhood that they know no other. When I am gone, they will whisper and tiptoe around, waiting for that crackly, tired voice to mutter,
Could you quiet down please? (I have always said *please*).
But that mutter won't be there. Eventually they will forget their inhibitions and they will learn to be children again. My husband won't have to sneak into the bedroom, using a flashlight to rummage through his dresser drawers. There will

be no one to disturb, no lump on the mattress.

I should take the Gravol at least an hour ahead. By then I will be sleepy anyway. Drowsy, unrushed, sedate. I will set myself against the base of a tree trunk. I will look up. The trees will form an enclosure, a secret garden, shielding me. I will not feel small or insignificant this time. I will meld into the essence of the forest. It will bless me, accept me.

I don't know how many of these pills I will need. Not many. Only one and I would be asleep within minutes. But awake again in an hour. I must swallow enough to keep me asleep until the nighttime temperatures drop below zero. Enough to render me incoherent should I wake. I will take them religiously, like communion. The bread and the wine. Likely, inside that huge god-shaped space within me, I will be praying. I will say,

Oh God, forgive me for I am a sinner.

It might be more astute of me to remove my boots, carry them across the river to the other side where they would be less likely to look for me. I would prefer not to be found, let the wild beasts have a scanty meal at least.

Then I will lie down. I should find a mossy area, my head elevated on an exposed root perhaps. Shall I curl up, hug my knees, bow my head? Or shall I lie with my arms behind my head, gazing up through the swaying canopy of trees? Likely there will be no clouds. The sky will be clear. My mind will be clear. The silence will no longer be turbulent. It will be empty. Not even empty, just quiet. Still. At last I shall have my stillness. It will almost be like crawling into my father's mushy lap and having all my insecurities vanish. Even now, though he is a doddering old man with wisps of white hair twisting sporadically around his temples, he would cuddle me and wrap his spotted arms around my bony shoulders and he would say,

You're not big enough to be grown up, Baby Doll. Aren't you ever going to grow up?

No, Father, I'm not, is what I would reply.

I never felt grown up. I thought if I were taller maybe I would have felt more grown up. If the distance from my eyes to the ground were more substantial, or if I didn't stumble and find my face in walls or in the earth I would have felt more grown up. Or if I had dressed in suits and heels and gone off every morning to some high-rise office or had my hair done once a week, or gotten pedicures, manicures, I might have felt more grown up. Or if my hands were bigger, stronger, more capable. If I'd been able to drink coffee and read the paper from front to back. Ah, but these, too, are only illusions, fragments of a lost life, speculations, as King Solomon would have said.

I will go gentle into that good night. I will have overcome the survival instinct.

shshshshshshshshshsh

But then there is always that ineradicable element of curiosity that compels me to give tomorrow another chance. It could be better. One never knows.

And that which does not kill me shall make me stronger, although I'm not sure I believe this. Does anyone?

"We tread lightly, as ghosts, upon this earth, wiping the blood of purgatory from our soles."

- Kathleen Gabriella Kelly, 2001

Acknowledgments

Thanks to all of my family for giving me a story to tell. I love every one of you, special in-laws and all. Thanks to Vimal for his patience and help with graphic design and typesetting. And thanks to my lap top which allows me to write lying down.

And to my friend, Wilma...where are you, Wilma? Call me.